HABITS
FOR
BETTER VISION

20 SCIENTIFICALLY PROVEN WAYS TO IMPROVE YOUR EYESIGHT NATURALLY

AILEEN YI FAN

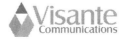

ISBN: 978-1-7332866-1-9 (Paperback)
ISBN: 978-1-7332866-0-2 (eBook)

Library of Congress Control Number: 2019909910

Book Cover Design: Danijela Mijailovic
Interior design: Lazar Kackarovski
Editor: Katie Chambers

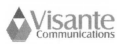

*To all readers who will
find this book useful.*

*To my children who inspired me
to write this book.*

TABLE OF CONTENTS

INTRODUCTION

My family story that begins the journey

William and Duncan, two brothers who grew up in China in the 1970s and 1980s, went to good (i.e., academically demanding) schools. At around age 14, both experienced myopia (nearsightedness), although they were diagnosed ten years apart because William is 10 years older than Duncan. Instead of turning to prescription glasses, they decided to try various ways to heal their vision naturally. They went outdoors and counted tree leaves during each 10-minute recess between 45-minute classes; they looked far away in the middle of reading or writing to relax their eyes; they exercised after school; they counted stars in the evening before bed; and they did various eye massages and drills throughout the day. Both kept their eyesight healthy and stable for the next few decades. As you might have guessed, William is my husband, and Duncan is my brother-in-law.

Fast forward three decades to the summer of 2014 when my son Ian had just turned nine years old. William took him to a regular pediatric ophthalmologist checkup before the new semester started, and Ian came back crying. The doctor told him that he had myopia and needed prescription glasses. Ian did not like that idea at all: he thought he would be teased by others; worse, his tennis "career" would be over if he wore glasses.

Somehow, I felt I had failed my son. Since our family had gone through major changes in 2013, I was so immersed in my own problems that I neglected taking care of him. I started researching natural cures on the internet, reading medical studies, buying books, and gathering anecdotal stories from friends and relatives. I was determined to help Ian. Together, we tried many different things to improve his eyesight naturally. Although the techniques were haphazardly applied, Ian maintained a good enough vision to navigate school, sports, and homework without prescription glasses for the past five years. Now I am revisiting this topic again because my 12-year-old daughter is facing the same challenge, mainly due to the heavy computer usage at both school and home.

Growing up in China, I was surrounded by myopic people. My parents and many of my teachers, relatives, and friends have myopia. When I turned 17, in order to prepare for the college entrance exam, I started boarding at my high school. Looking back, it was ultimately a bad decision. I studied for long hours in dim-lit classrooms without any outdoor time or physical activities. I had horrible nutrition intake and had problems falling asleep in a dormitory with seven other girls—all in a stressful time preparing for the exam that can make or break a child's dream. Within four months, my 20/15 vision quickly deteriorated to 20/70. On the night I saw a big halo around the full moon, I silently cried for the whole night. In the following years, my prescription glasses increased by −0.25 diopters each time I got new glasses until I hit −3.25 diopters. When I stopped going to optometrists to get new glasses, my eyesight actually stabilized. The trend started to reverse slowly after my studying this topic. I wish I had the current me with the knowledge, wisdom, and determination to support the helpless 17-year-old me.

The myopia epidemic

Myopia affected approximately 1.6 billion people worldwide in 2000, and that statistic is expected to increase to 2.5 billion by 2020,[1] and to nearly 5 billion by 2050.[2] The prevalence of myopia in the developed countries of East and Southeast Asia increased from about 10–30 percent to 80–90 percent in young adults.[3] According to the National Eye Institute (NEI), about 42 percent of Americans ages 12–54 are nearsighted, up from 25 percent in 1971. In Western Europe, the described prevalence was 26.6 percent. Children from urban environments are more than twice as likely to be myopic than those from rural environments. Researchers frequently report that near work (such as reading, writing, time looking at a screen, etc.), education, age, economic status, and height are associated with myopia.

Some doctors believe myopia is hereditary, but myopia is virtually non-existent in pre-industrialized cultures. Plus, gene pools cannot possibly change fast enough to affect 1 billion more people (which is a 56 percent increase) in just a short 20-year period. Studies carried out in hunter-gatherer societies and in recently westernized hunter-gatherer groups indicate that myopia normally occurs in 0 to 2 percent of the population, and moderate to high myopia is either non-existent or occurs in about one person out of 1,000. Thus, the prevalence of myopia today is increasing so fast that environmental and social factors must be involved. The epidemic of blurred vision can be traced back to physical, mental, emotional, and spiritual imbalances of our modern society.

Although most myopia cases can be corrected by optics or surgery, normal and high myopia are still unsolved medical problems. Studies indicate that myopia is a major factor behind vision impairment and blindness in adults. It frequently predisposes people, especially those who have myopia of -6D or worse (in which objects appear blurred when they are 16–17 cm or 6–7 in away), to suffer from other eye pathologies such as retinal detachment, glaucoma, macular hemorrhage, cataracts, and so on.

Why did I write this book?

Chances are that you, like many of us today, tend to have a sedentary lifestyle. We also engage in too much close work—reading, writing, using computer screens and smart phones—but far less outdoor activities. Too much close work causes eye strain and muscle spasms, which give us blurry distance vision (myopic symptoms). Instead of addressing the root cause of muscle spasm and related mental strain, medical professionals prescribe glasses and contact lenses to give us a quick and easy fix. But this easy fix often progressively worsens the eyesight as the eyes become trained to work within the confines of the lenses. In addition, glasses are stimuli to our eyes; as a result, our eyes grow longer axially, and we become chronically dependent on prescription lenses.

Many vision coaches, classes, and online teachings help people reverse myopia, but they are neither accepted nor recommended by mainstream doctors. Yet many of these teachings produce good results even though they are not quick and easy fixes, because myopia has complicated causes and requires many facets of lifestyle, belief, mind, body, and habitual changes.

Our eyes are not broken, and our genes are not problematic. We have the power to form new habits to improve our eyesight, starting right now and right away. We are so much more powerful to heal ourselves than we believe we are. With this book, I hope to plant a seed of self-empowerment not only to help you improve your eyesight, but also to gain the "spill over" effect in your general health and well-being.

This book has taken me five years to write since my first impulse in 2014. In it, I distill the information I learned from numerous sources; combine my research of nutritional studies and experiments at home; and discuss the mind, body, and spiritual studies I conducted over the past several years. I sincerely hope this book can increase the public awareness of natural and integrated eye care.

I had doubted my authority, but I have a mission to bring this information to parents and children who may not have the time or knowledge to do the research. I aspire to bring hope and love to these people who suffer or lose any kind of freedom due to myopia.

How do you use this book?

John F. Kennedy said, "The time to repair a roof is when the sun is shining." Perhaps you are fortunate enough not to have any vision problems. I just want to remind you that the time to prevent myopia is when your eyesight is good. Don't take your vision for granted. Your eyes make the intricate and incredible conversion of light to sight—it is indeed miraculous. Don't wait to nurture your vision, do it today.

Perhaps you had started wearing glasses and missed the most precious opportunity to reverse your myopia, but do not lose hope. I encourage you to form new eye care habits listed in the book, and you will not only stop worsening myopia, but also get a chance to reverse it if you are committed to these habits.

With that said, this book is not a one-size-fits-all solution for your vision. You can choose to implement what applies to you, use what works for you, or start from the easiest steps such as hanging a $10 Snellen chart at home, removing the night-light from your bedroom, and relaxing your eyes more frequently during close work. Small habitual changes can produce remarkable long-term results. Some changes are more difficult, like engaging in more outdoor activities and reducing screen time. Your diet change is likely another. But as the old adage goes, "the journey of a thousand miles begins with a single step." This book can be a resource to support and encourage you to start that single step towards your journey of natural vision improvement.

If you are a parent who picked up this book, congratulations! You now can help your child either prevent or improve myopia with this new knowledge. I hope this book can support you just like I supported my children who are going through this experience right now.

With love,

Aileen

What Is Myopia?

MYOPIA IS ALSO KNOWN as nearsightedness. According to the NEI,[1] myopia occurs when the eye grows too long from front to back (axially). Instead of focusing images on the retina—the light-sensitive tissue in the back of the eye—the lens of the myopic eye focuses the image in front of the retina. In a normal eye, the light focuses on the retina. Myopia also can be the result of a cornea—the eye's outermost layer—that is too curved for the length of the eyeball or a lens that is too thick.

People with myopia have good near vision but poor distance vision; they can typically see well enough to read a book or computer screen but struggle to see objects farther away. Sometimes people with undiagnosed myopia have headaches and eyestrain from struggling to clearly see things in the distance. In medical terms, myopia is simply a refractive state, not a disease, that causes distant objects to appear blurry.

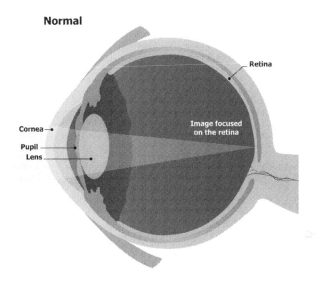

Figure 1 *The normal eye*

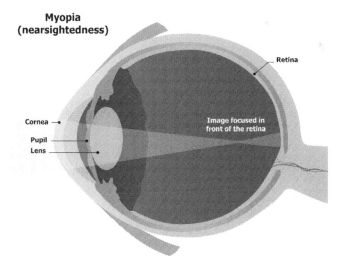

Figure 2 *The myopic eye*

What causes myopia?

According to NEI, genetics plays a role in myopia. But the recent dramatic increase in the prevalence of myopia around the world points to environmental causes such as lack of time spent outdoors, and greater amount of time spent doing near work. Based on my research, other factors that cause myopia include eye-muscle fatigue, mental stress and strain, insufficient exposure to sunlight, inadequate sleep, inadequate nutrition, long periods of wearing glasses or contacts, bad posture, and lack of mental focus. Most of these factors are features of our modern lifestyle. It is safe to say myopia is caused by the combined body, mind, and environmental factors.

How is myopia diagnosed?

According to the American Academy of Ophthalmology (AAO),[2] Myopia is often discovered when children are between the ages of eight and twelve. Children may complain of headaches, rub their eyes, squint frequently, perform poorly in school, trip, or seem clumsy.

An eye care professional can diagnose myopia during a comprehensive eye exam, which includes testing vision and examining the eye in detail. When possible, an eye exam should include the use of dilating eye drops to open the pupils wide for close examination of the optic nerve and retina. Going to an ophthalmologist's office for your initial exam would be more recommended than a store that sells glasses or contact lenses. This is because in most cases (but not all), the length of the exam and the incentive of the professionals will be different in the two locations.

How is myopia corrected?

According to eye care professionals, the most common way to treat myopia is with corrective eyeglasses or contact lenses, which refocus light onto the retina. Refractive surgery is an option only for adults who meet certain criteria. According to the NEI, both contact lenses and refractive surgery can cause complications. Additionally, none of these corrections improve the underlying condition of myopia. They only treat the symptom, not the causes. With this book, I encourage you to prevent or stop your myopia progression through natural and integrated eye care.

What is pseudomyopia?

Children usually start with pseudomyopia, also known as NITM (near induced transient myopia). This is what happened to William, Duncan, and Ian when they first had their myopia symptoms. While this condition is similar to myopia—the eye can see near objects clearly, but the distance objects appear blurry—it is more of a temporary condition from long periods of time in close work. The ciliary muscles (the focusing muscles of the eye) undergo spasms and cannot unwind even when the eyes are looking at a distance—when these muscles are supposed to relax. Rest can solve the problem, but continued overuse can lead to a further loss of distance vision. At this stage, the eyeballs have not yet grown longer axially, so the myopia is not permanent.

What is progressive myopia/ lens-induced myopia?

Myopia progression is typically associated with axial elongation.[3] When pseudomyopic children are given prescription glasses, they regain their distance vision immediately. Happy with this quick fix, they continue with their bad habits. But the real cause—overused eye muscles—is not fixed. Wearing glasses creates a stimulus to the eye because the glasses change the eye's focal plane. The eyes are designed to correct their length according to the new stimulus. As a result, the eyes grow longer axially and pseudomyopia becomes progressive myopia, also called lens-induced myopia.

The normal axial length of a human eyeball is approximately 24–25 millimeters.[5] A one-millimeter elongation of axial length without other compensation is equivalent to a myopic shift of −2 or −2.5 diopters.[6]

What to do when myopia symptoms first show up?

I know how a parent feels when being told "your child needs glasses" for the first time. In my son's case, instead of getting glasses, we immediately started with the eye exercises, sunshine, outdoors, and the evening routines stated in this book. We did prepare a pair of glasses for him just in case, but he has not used the glasses at all.

I would recommend you do the same—start reading this book and make a plan to reverse the pseudomyopia. If your child needs a pair of glasses to see well in the classroom, remember to teach them the habit of using the glasses only for distance vision (see habit #9).

What is visual acuity?

Visual acuity refers to the clarity or sharpness of vision, measured by the ability to discern letters or numbers at a given distance according to a fixed standard. Normal visual acuity is 20/20. If you have 20/20 vision, you can see clearly at 20 feet (6 meters) what should normally be seen at that distance. If you have 20/100 vision, it means that you must be as close as 20 feet to see what a person with normal vision can see at 100 feet. To measure visual acuity, you can use a Snellen chart.

According to American Optometric Association (AOA), having 20/20 vision does not necessarily mean you have perfect vision. This only indicates the sharpness or clarity of vision at a distance. Other important vision skills—such as peripheral awareness or side vision, eye coordination, depth perception, focus ability, and color vision—all contribute to your overall visual ability.

What are diopters?

A diopter is the power of the lens needed to correct the vision back to normal (20/20). Zero diopter is 20/20; the higher the number, the stronger the lens. The Khan Academy's video "Diopters, Aberration, and the Human Eye"[4] explains how to calculate diopters:

Diopter = 1 ÷ Distance to blur
(measured in meter [m])

For example, if the furthest distance you can read a word clearly on a page is 20 inches (0.5 meters), then the diopter number would be 2.0 (1÷ 0.5). Myopia uses negative lens, so the diopter would be –2.0.

Jake Steiner from Endmyopia.org[6] simplified the diopter calculation so you can measure it easily at home: (1) Read the text on the screen until it just barely starts to blur. (2) Measure the distance (in meters) from your eyes to the screen, aka "Distance to blur." (3) Calculate the diopter using the formula: Diopter = 1 ÷ Distance to blur (measured in meters).

What is low, moderate, and high myopia?

One of the classifications of myopia is low, moderate, and high myopia with the following criteria.[7]

- Low myopia: less than –3 diopters, which means the distance to blur is about 13 inches (0.33 m) from the eye. The roughly estimated visual acuity is 20/150 or better.

- Moderate myopia: between –3 and –6 diopters, which means the distance to blur is between 6–7 inches (0.17 m) to 13 inches (0.33 m). The estimated visual acuity is about 20/150 to 20/500.

- High myopia: anything above –6 diopters, which means the distance to blur is less than 6–7 inches (0.17 m). The estimated visual acuity is below 20/500.

PART I: Belief

*"Whether you think you can,
or you think you can't—you're right."*

~Henry Ford ~

*"Drugs are not always necessary.
Belief in recovery always is."*

~Norman Cousins ~

HABIT #1
Change Your Beliefs

Henry Ford's quote applies to your eyesight too—whether you believe you can improve your eyesight, or you believe you can't—you're right. In habit #1, you will learn to challenge your belief that myopia is irreversible. Let's empower you to reverse your pseudomyopia or even myopia if you are committed to it. In my research of this book, I have come across many natural vision improvement coaches and numerous success stories.

We are wired to follow what we believe is true. Some even say our thoughts and beliefs create our reality. However, a belief is just the thought we repeatedly think. Some of them serve us, some of them don't, so it is worth letting go of the ones that don't support us. We can make changes, starting with changing our thoughts and beliefs.

I want to share with you two exciting studies that support myopia reversal. In April 2013, the *Journal of Investigative Ophthalmology & Visual Science (IOVS)* published a remarkable study, titled "Various Species Can Shorten to Compensate for Myopic Defocus."[1] The research scientists demonstrated that the eyes of young animals of four various species (chick, tree shrew, marmoset, and rhesus macaque) can shorten in the axial dimension in response to myopic defocus. They also concluded that the implications for human myopia control are significant. This is fundamental to the myopia reversal theory because it proves that the axial changes can go both ways—elongation (myopia) or shortening (reversal of myopia).

Another motivating study "Human Optical Axial Length and Defocus"[2] revealed significant changes in optical axial length in human after 60 minutes of monocular defocus. Researchers studied 28 young adults (half with myopia and half with perfect vision) with four different monocular (only one eye) defocus conditions. The study proved that bidirectional optical axial length changes do happen—i.e., axial changes go both ways—in response to defocus. Thus, this suggests that the human visual system can detect the presence and sign of defocus, and change optical axial length to move the retina toward the image plane. The researchers gave clinical evidence that distinctive axial changes in human eyes can happen in as little as 60 minutes! Now we have the hope to cure the so-called "incurable" myopia.

Dr. Bruce Lipton, stem cell biologist and a pioneer in epigenetics, states that around one percent of disease is due to genetic aberrations, which means more than 90 percent of life's dysfunctions are attributed to environmental stressors. Our perceptions, beliefs, and responses to stressors determine our state of health or disease.[3]

For some, a strong belief that a treatment will heal an ailment can prompt the brain to tap into its own pharmacy, flooding the nervous system with medicating neurotransmitters and hormones. The power of a positive belief is recognized by science as an expression of the "placebo effect"—one third of all participants in drug trials experience the positive healing credited to a medication although they only received the equivalent of a sugar pill. What exactly healed these people? The answer is the power of positive thinking! What's even more thought-provoking is the "nocebo effect," which also happens in the drug trials. This effect occurs when the participants who receive sugar pills show side effects of a drug such as dizziness, vomiting, headaches, and other life-threatening symptoms. It is not the sugar pill that caused side effects; it is the power of negative beliefs!

Dr. Ellen Warner pointed out in her article in the *Canadian Medical Association Journal* "The Role of Belief in Healing"[4] that modern technological medicine may occasionally cure disease but will never heal the patient. When the topic "why do people get well?" arose, the answer was "neuropeptides," "belief," "behavior modification.". . . More and more holistic medical professionals are embracing the mind-body connection and encouraging us to modify our beliefs, emotions, behaviors, and habits to heal our bodies, including our precious eyes.

Martin Sussman, the founder of Cambridge Institute for Better Vision, has helped hundreds of thousands of people to improve their vision naturally since the 1970s. In his book, *The Program for Better Vision. How to See Better in Minutes a Day without Glasses or Contacts,*[5] he stated that the way we see reflects who we are, and how we respond to life situations. Improving our eyesight is a process of self-discovery, learning, and growth. It provides an opportunity for us to broaden our perspective, improve our self-image, gain emotional clarity, and focus our energy and concentration more effectively.

Louise Hay, a motivational author and the founder of Hay House Publishing company, is known for empowering people to unleash the doctor/healer within each of us. In her book *You can Heal Your Life*[6] which has sold more than 50 million copies worldwide, Louise cited that the probable causes of myopia are fear of the future and not trusting what's ahead. She encourages us to do several things: (1) look up the possible mental cause, (2) repeat "I am willing to release the pattern in my consciousness that has created this condition," (3) repeatedly use new thought patterns such as "I trust the process of life. I am safe," (4) assume we are already in the process of healing our eyesight.

I truly hope these studies and books bring hope and create a mental shift in you—that you can do something good for your eyes and improve your eyesight. This is the foundation of healing.

ACTION STEPS

Write this affirmation on a card and read it every morning:

Today, I affirm that I am empowered to make changes and do something good for my vision. My eyesight is simply a refractive state, not a defect, illness, or error. Scientific studies have shown that the eye axial changes can go both ways, and so can my eyes. I am willing to release the pattern in my consciousness that has created my condition. I trust the process of life. I am safe. Today I am committed to doing something good for my eyes. I am willing to learn how to relax and reactivate my vision. I am already in the process of healing.

HABIT #2

Take Caution of Quick Fixes

OUR CULTURE LOVES INSTANT gratification and quick fixes. Modern technology causes us to lose patience even more, demanding we find a solution right away. When myopia symptoms show up, prescription lenses are usually the first recommendation by medical professionals—to help us regain distant vision immediately. Then we can continue our bad habits as usual.

I was doing the same after becoming a myope myself. I visited the optometrist office every year or every other year. Almost every visit, I got a new pair of more powerful glasses, usually –0.25 or –0.5 diopter worse. I always felt dizzy with new glasses because they make everything look different, so my eyes have to adapt each time. Soon I got used to the new glasses, which means my eyes grew a little longer to adapt to these higher power glasses; thus, I developed progressive myopia. When my insurance company dropped the coverage, I stopped visiting the optometrist office. To my delight, my eyesight stabilized for many years, and I could see everything I needed to see with my existing glasses. With my new research, I started to reverse myopia slowly but gradually, as I had 30 years of glass wearing history. Today, I wear my old glasses I had more than 15 years ago, and I only wear them when I drive or need to see things clearly in the distance.

We know glasses only address the symptom but do not cure myopia. Dr. William H. Bates, an ophthalmologist from the early 20th century, was the pioneer of myopia prevention and natural vision improvement.[1] He noticed that the eye muscles have constant mild strain while one is wearing low prescription glasses and quite a lot of strain while one is wearing high prescription glasses. And since you must constantly recreate the strain you had while getting fitted for the glasses, your eyes are under a lot of strain when you wear them. So, to give your eyes space to relax, you will want to take the glasses off whenever it is feasible and safe.

Pseudomyopia

Children always start with pseudomyopia, or NITM. It is caused by the spasm of ciliary muscles through engaging in too much near work. With pseudomyopia, the eyeball has not yet grown longer. The most effective treatment is to fully relax the muscles and reverse the muscle spasm. (Habit #7, #8 and #12 provide many ways to relax the eye muscles). Studies have shown atropine in extremely low concentration could significantly slow myopia progression in children.[2] Atropine is often used before eye examinations to fully relax eye muscles. However, atropine requires professional involvement, and the studies are mostly documented in Asian countries.

Progressive myopia

After people begin to wear glasses, the power of the lenses, in most cases, has to be steadily increased, and the vision gets worse progressively. Doug Marsh quoted optometrist Joseph Kennebeck in his book *Restoring Your Eyesight*: "Glasses are prescribed for one distance—twenty feet . . . looking through the lenses at objects closer than 20 feet means the eyes have to overaccommodate (unnaturally strain to adjust focus) because glasses are too strong for close work . . . At TEN feet, the glasses are TWICE wrong; at FIVE feet the glasses are FOUR times wrong; at ONE foot, the glasses are TWENTY times wrong. The eyes cannot compensate . . . without being HURT. It is the compensating, through myopic glasses fitted for 20 feet, that brings on progressive myopia, or lens-induced myopia."[3]

The debate between under-correction and full correction

Under-correction refers to a myope getting a pair of prescription glasses that gives a distance acuity of 20/40, instead of the full correction of 20/20. The corrective lens has slightly lower power than required (i.e., 0.50 diopter less than the full-strength correction). For example, if an eye's full correction is –2.00 diopters, the under-corrected prescription would be –1.50 diopters. It means with the glasses, you will see good enough, but not super clear at a distance.

The studies that support under-correction included animal studies on monkeys and chicks,[4-5] and the 2017 Chinese children study.[6] Animal studies have demonstrated that the eye will adjust its growth in response to visual stimulus, with axial growth accelerated when the ocular image is focused behind the retina and slowed when focused in front of the retina. Following this logic, under-correction shifts the ocular image in front of the retina, thus, slowing down axial growth and myopia progression.

In a 2017 study titled "Effect of Under-correction Versus Full Correction on Myopia Progression in 12-year-old Children,"[6] the researchers from China investigated the effects of no correction against full correction to assess myopia progression. One hundred and twenty myopic children with an average age of 12.7 years were involved in a two-year research. Like the animal studies, at the two-year follow-up, myopia progression reduced significantly with an increasing amount of under-correction in all children. Children with no correction had slower myopia progression and less axial elongation than children with full correction. The uncorrected children progressed by –0.75 diopter over two years, while the fully corrected children progressed by –1.04 diopters.

To add controversy, a 2012 study "Under-correction of Myopia Increases Myopic Progression—A Retrospective Study"[7] found under-correction of myopia produced a greater degree of myopic progression than did full correction in children and young adults. The study was based on patient records of a private optometric practice in Arizona with 78 people from 6–35 years, among them 42 children under 18 years old.

No matter what side you choose, remember glasses tend to do more harm than good, and at their best, they never improve the vision to normal. If you have to get glasses, find a professional who supports under-correction and read habit #9 to learn how to use prescription glasses.

ACTION STEPS

○ Before you get your first pair of prescription glasses, read this book and decide to make the habitual changes outlined in the future chapters.

○ You can get glasses but remember to only use them for distance vision. Ask the doctor to prescribe corrective lens with slightly lower power than required.

○ Take off the glasses when you are doing near work such as reading, writing, or working on a computer or other electronic devices.

○ Use glasses less than two to three hours a day if you can.

PART II: Body

*"Health is a state of complete mental,
social and physical well-being, not merely
the absence of disease or infirmity."*

~ *World Health Organization, 1948* ~

*"The doctor of the future will give no medicine
but will instruct his patients in care of the human frame,
in diet, and in the cause and prevention of disease."*

~ *Thomas Edison* ~

HABIT #3
Examine Your Lifestyle

LIFESTYLE REFERS TO THE way individuals, families, and societies live. It is expressed in work, study, and leisure behavior patterns in activities, attitudes, interests, opinions, values, and income allocation. While our modern lifestyle provides many advantages, such as using modern machines to make life easier, more productive, more comfortable, easier to stay connected, and easier to access education, our unique culture and tradition are fading off and people are becoming addicted to technology and material life. We have constant stimulus from the internet, the news, social media, video games, smartphones, and numerous electronic gadgets. In fact, according to a new study by Nielsen, a market-research company, American adults spend more than 11 hours per day watching, reading, listening to, or simply interacting with media.

Our life has become fast-paced and stressful, and we have less free time to spend outdoors and pay undivided attention to our family and friends. We are living in the busiest period in history; the speed of life has increased exponentially over the past 100 years, while the evolution of our body, brain, and eyes have not.

The alarming statistics of myopia

Because of this lifestyle change, myopia has become an epidemic in many parts of the world.[1] In addition to the 41.6 percent of Americans who are nearsighted, the myopia rate in young Americans is estimated as high as 60 percent.[2] "The trend appears to be upwards in many other parts of the world, but the changes have been nowhere near as spectacular as in East and Southeast Asia," said Ian Morgan, Ph.D., a renowned myopia researcher at Australian National University. In the developed countries of East and Southeast Asia, the prevalence has now reached 80 to 90 percent among children with 12 years of school.[3,4]

Projections suggest that almost 50 percent of the world will be myopic by 2050. The May 2016 issue of *Ophthalmology* published a study called "Global Prevalence of Myopia and High Myopia and Temporal Trends from 2000 through 2050"[5] where the researchers analyzed data from 145 studies covering 2.1 million participants. They discovered that increases in myopia are driven principally by lifestyle, particularly by the increased time on near-work activities, often electronic devices. More and more schools are adopting digital education systems, making it impossible to limit the electronic devices to balance the child's school days. As a result, more and more children are wearing glasses.

The other research published in *JAMA Ophthalmology* named "Myopia, Lifestyle, and Schooling in Students of Chinese Ethnicity in Singapore and Sydney"[6] studied the prevalence and risk factors of myopia in six- and seven-year-old children of Chinese ethnicity in Sydney and Singapore. The researchers concluded that myopia in Chinese ethnicity was significantly lower in Sydney (3.3 percent) than in Singapore (29.1 percent). In Sydney, children read more books per week and did more total near-work activities, but they also spend more time outdoors. But Singapore children have less outdoor activities and much higher early educational pressures.

Electronic devices and the blue light

Until the advent of artificial lighting, the sun was the major source of blue light. However, with the growth of technology, LED screens—computer monitors, smart phones, tablets, and LED TV—are now becoming the number one source of blue light. The 380–420 nm short blue light waves from these devices are harmful to human eyes. According to a NEI-funded study, children's eyes absorb more blue light than adults from digital device screens.

Not all children who do their homework on a PC and tablet develop myopia, but if they do, the blue light from those screens must have played some role in it. Parents and teachers must be aware of the usage and control the children's total time on screens on a given day. This includes school usage, homework, and games.

The sedentary lifestyle

In the US and around the world, people are spending more and more time doing sedentary activities. Many of us sit in front of the computer at work; sit during our leisure time to watch TV, engage in social media, or games; then we sit more in cars, buses, or flights. The US National Library of Medicine warns that a sedentary lifestyle has many health risks—it causes us to gain weight, waste away muscles, weaken our bones, compromise our immune systems, and have poorer blood circulation. Many chronic diseases such as diabetes, obesity, high blood pressure, cancer, and even depression are the results of this inactive lifestyle.[7]

Although not a disease, myopia as a common type of refractive error is also a byproduct of the modern inactive lifestyle. In a study published in *IVOS* "Risk Factors for Childhood Myopia: Findings from the NICER Study,"[8] researchers from Northern Ireland evaluated risk factors for myopia in 12- to 13-year-old white children. The data showed that regular physical activity was associated with a lower estimated prevalence of myopia compared to sedentary lifestyles.

To prevent or reverse myopia, we must change our inactive lifestyle right away. The first step is perhaps to follow the recommendation from an ex-NASA employee Dr. Joan Vernikos. Dr. Vernikos said our physical health is not determined by how long we stand or how long we sit, but rather the number of times we alternate positions. She recommends going from a sitting to standing position at least 25 times per day.

NIH calls sedentary lifestyle "a sitting disease." It is time for us to choose a conscious and healthy lifestyle. As the old saying goes, "health is wealth"; good health lets us enjoy life and manage its challenges, and most importantly enjoy our healthy vision. Remember our body is one integrated system rather than a collection of independent organs. In order to identify and address the root causes of myopia, we need a whole health protocol—to heal the mind-body-spirit through a new lifestyle that improves the overall wellness of our body.

ACTION STEPS

- Limit TV, electronic devices, and computer usage to as little time as possible.

- Increase time spent outdoors, including physical activities and unstructured play in nature.

○ Be more active indoors. Remember to go from a sitting to a standing position at least 25 times per day. To be more active around the house, you can clean your room, make your bed, or just stand up and move around every 20–30 minutes.

○ Schedule quality time to connect with family and friends in person with undivided attention instead of connected on social media.

HABIT #4

Eat a Nutrient-Rich Diet

ALTHOUGH THE BRAIN IS only 2 percent of our body weight, it uses 20 to 30 percent of the nutritional intake and 20 percent of the oxygen intake—more than any other human organ. The visual system is an energetically demanding system in the brain because the retina has one of the highest metabolic needs of the body—it consumes as much as 25 percent of the nutrition and 35 percent of the oxygen the brain takes.

We must ensure that our eyes get the nutrients they need because more than 80 percent of what we learn about this world is through our eyes. Our eyesight is a complex function that extends from the eyes to the optic nerves and occipital lobe (the visual processing center) inside our brain. The optic nerve is the only place where the brain meets the outside world. Dr. Neal Adams, an ophthalmologist, sees the eyes as the window to the body. The back of the eye can be the first place he sees signs of diabetes, high blood pressure, and even cancer.

Good nutrition is an important part of brain health and eye health. In today's fast-food-, boxed food-, and processed food-dominated culture, many of us are overfed but undernourished. We are depriving ourselves of live and natural nutrients that are imperative to the proper functioning of our body and our eyes. That is why health-conscious people call the standard American diet SAD.

There is a deep connection between our food and our eyes: what we eat can nourish or damage our eye health. However, we don't get proper nutrition education in school; even doctors don't study nutrition in medical schools. The good news is that mainstream medicine is starting to embrace nutrition and health, as we are seeing more and more studies in this area.

The *Ophthalmology* journal recently published a study by the Eye-Risk Consortium called "Mediterranean Diet and Incidence of Advanced Age-Related Macular Degeneration."[1] Dr. Emily Chew, a clinical spokesperson for the American Academy of Ophthalmology, who serves on an advisory board to the research group said, "You are what you eat. I believe this is a public health issue on the same scale as smoking. Chronic diseases such as AMD (Age-Related Macular Degeneration), dementia, obesity, and diabetes, all have roots in poor dietary habits. It's time to take quitting a poor diet as seriously as quitting smoking." It is time for us to educate ourselves in nutrition.

Nourishing whole foods

In general, the eyes and body benefit from a whole food diet (consisting of naturally grown foods). The word diet here does not refer to a weight loss attempt or program, but simply means you decide what you will eat today. The whole foods diet includes a broad variety of nutrients and micronutrients that interact and support each other in a balanced and harmonious way. The Eye-Risk Consortium studied 4,500 French and Dutch adults, and found that a diet rich in healthful nutrient-rich foods, such as fruits, vegetables, legumes, and fish, plays a key role in the prevention of a variety of chronic diseases including eye diseases. Also eating a rainbow variety of fresh food is vital for optimal brain and eye health. The red, orange, yellow, green, blue, and purple variation of fruits and vegetables offer vitamins, minerals, antioxidants, and phytochemicals—all of which have enormous healing powers.

Since a type of omega-3 fatty acid called DHA (docosahexaenoic acid) makes up half of the fats in the brain and retina, we need to eat more fish high in omega-3, such as salmon, sardine, and mackerel; and seeds such as flaxseed, chia seed, and hemp seed. On the other hand, omega-6 fatty acids, prevalent in highly processed vegetable oils, may increase the risk of chronic diseases.

The researchers also found that none of the components of a Mediterranean diet—fish, fruit, vegetables, nuts, and seeds—lowered the risk of age-related macular degeneration on their own. Rather, it was the entire pattern of eating a nutrient-rich diet that reduced the risk significantly.[1]

Antioxidants and phytochemicals

In the research article "Oxidative Stress in Myopia,"[2] the researchers found that oxidative stress is part of the molecular basis that is associated with myopia. Oxidative stress occurs when you have an imbalance between free radical production and antioxidant defense. These free radicals come from natural by-products from the body's metabolic processes and immune responses, and from fried foods, drugs, alcohol, tobacco, pesticides, and air pollutants. They can cause damage to parts of cells, such as proteins, DNA, and cell membranes, resulting in diseases.

Antioxidants are "free radical scavengers" that either reduce the formation of free radicals or neutralize them. These micronutrients act as significant protective factors. For example, dietary carotenoids are thought to provide health benefits in decreasing the risk of disease, particularly certain cancers and eye diseases. The carotenoids that have been most studied are beta-carotene, lycopene, lutein, and zeaxanthin.[3]

Benefits of antioxidants to the eye

- Lycopene: protects against oxidative damage to lipids, proteins, and DNA. It helps reduce the risk of macular degeneration and cataracts later in life.

- Lutein and zeaxanthin: absorb blue light, defend free radicals, and prevent many age-related eye diseases.

- Flavonoids: improve night vision and eye health, and lower the risks of cataracts, macular degeneration, and other chronic diseases.

- Glutathione: stimulates immune system and prevents human myopic cataracts.

- Vitamin A (or beta-carotene, vitamin A's precursor): improves general eye health and night vision and lowers the risk of cataracts and macular degeneration later in life.

- Vitamin C: helps reduce chronic diseases, strengthens the immune system, repairs and regenerates tissues, and reduces the risk of cataracts and macular degeneration later in life.

- Vitamin E: helps maintain good eyesight and reduces the risk of cataracts and macular degeneration later in life.

Foods that are rich in these helpful antioxidants

- Lycopene: fruits and vegetables with red and pink pigments, such as tomato, watermelon, red orange, pink grapefruit, apricot, rosehip, and guava.

- Lutein and zeaxanthin: pumpkin, carrot, citrus fruits, and egg yolk.

- Flavonoids: many fruits and vegetables, especially berries and grapes.

- Glutathione: asparagus, avocado, broccoli, garlic, onions, spinach, tomato, watermelon, egg, and walnut. Be aware that acetaminophen (Tylenol) decreases intracellular glutathione levels,[4] so it is not a good pain reliever for anyone concerned with eye health.

- Vitamin A (or beta-carotene, A's precursor): citrus fruits, melons, carrot, spinach, broccoli, and animal liver or cod liver oil.

- Vitamins C: citrus fruits, berries, melons, carrot, peppers, and leafy green vegetables.

- Vitamin E: beets, broccoli, leafy greens, whole grains, sunflower seeds, and almonds.

Phytochemicals, naturally occurring compounds in plant foods such as fruits, vegetables, whole grains, beans, nuts and seeds, can act as antioxidants, neutralizing free radicals and removing their power to create damage. For example, overwhelming evidence has shown that berry fruits have beneficial effects against human cancers. They also counteract, reduce, and repair damages from oxidative stress and inflammation. The anticancer and anti-inflammatory potential of berries is related to a multitude of bioactive phytochemicals including polyphenols (flavonoids, proanthocyanidins, ellagitannins, gallotannins, phenolic acids), stilbenoids, lignans, and triterpenoids.[5]

Vitamins and minerals

According to the NIH National Center for Complementary and Integrative Health, vitamins and minerals are essential substances that our bodies need to develop and function normally. The known essential vitamins include A, C, D, E, K, and the B vitamins: thiamin (B1), riboflavin (B2), niacin (B3), pantothenic acid (B5), pyridoxal (B6), cobalamin (B12), biotin, and folate/folic acid.

We also need minerals for our health: calcium, phosphorus, potassium, sodium, chloride, magnesium, iron, zinc, iodine, sulfur, cobalt, copper, fluoride, manganese, and selenium. For example, the study "Prevention of Axial Elongation in Myopia by the Trace Element Zinc,"[6] revealed that zinc can inhibit the axial elongation of the eye and can be used to prevent and treat myopia to a certain extent. Certain meats, seafood, seeds, and beans are rich in zinc.

The 2015–2020 Dietary Guidelines for Americans recommends that people should aim to meet their nutrient requirements through a healthy eating pattern that includes nutrient-dense forms of foods.[7] *Nature* magazine's well-known article "Nutrition Supplements and the Eye"[8] also provides a review of the roles of vitamins, minerals, carotenoids, and essential fatty acids in relation to eye health. It summarizes what we discussed above—vital nutrients, healthy fat, vitamins, and trace minerals are important in retinal development and preventing eye diseases. They also promote bodily health on which the eye depends.

Avoid processed food, not just for the eye

A large study published in the *British Journal of Psychiatry* found eating processed foods, such as refined carbohydrates, sweets, and processed meats, increased the risk of depression by about 60 percent. Eating a whole foods diet, on the other hand, decreased the risk by about 26 percent.[9] In another study published in the *British Medical Journal*, the researchers found that an increase in the proportion of ultra-processed foods in the diet was associated with significantly increased risks of cancer.[10]

Do your body and eyes a big favor and avoid the toxic foods that create chronic inflammation: all forms of refined carbohydrates, refined sugar, sugary drinks, refined vegetable oils, and highly processed foods that come in a box, a can, or a bag. For example, unlike marine-based omega-3 fat, omega-6 fat found in refined vegetable oils are oxidized and can be toxic. Artificial

sweeteners and genetically modified organisms (GMO)
are sensitive topics these days, but more and more
scientific studies are showing great concerns over them.
Processed and packaged foods contain preservatives,
which are chemicals that can pose a number of serious
health risks. Artificial flavors contained in many
processed foods decreases the amount of Vitamin C
in the body. Processed meat (which involves salting,
curing, fermenting, and smoking) was classified as
carcinogenic to humans (IARC Group 1) by the World
Health Organization (WHO). The IARC classifications
describe the strength of the scientific evidence about an
agent being a cause of cancer.[11] Thus, you should avoid
them as much as you can.

Sugar and refined carbohydrates such as breads,
cereals, cookies, and cakes increase the body's insulin
levels, which acts as a powerful stimulator of axial
myopia growth in animal and human studies. According
to Evolutionary Biologist Loren Cordain, higher insulin
levels affect the development of the eyeball, making it
abnormally long and causing nearsightedness. In his
study "An evolutionary Analysis of the Aetiology and
Pathogenesis of Juvenile-Onset Myopia,"[12] Cordain
found that when the hunter-gatherer societies change
their lifestyle and introduce grains and carbohydrates,
they rapidly develop (within a single generation) myopia
at rates that equal or exceed those in western societies.

In Dr. Ben Lane's research, "Calcium, Chromium,
Protein, Sugar and Accommodation in Myopia,"[13] he

found myopes, as a class, whether or not their myopia is increasing, are statistically deficient in chromium, and white sugar depletes chromium. Remember, refined sugar has more than 60 different names in food labels. The common names are sugar, sucrose, high-fructose corn syrup, corn syrup, barley malt, dextrose, maltose, and rice syrups, etc. Sugar is hidden in almost all processed foods including ketchups and yogurt. Soft drinks, juice, and sports drinks are all high in sugar. Sugar and refined carbohydrates give our body nutritional stress by depleting minerals, vitamins, and quality fats; thus, we are left with no protection against stress.

Michael Pollan, an author of several New York Times bestselling books on nutrition, points out that real food is alive—and therefore should eventually die (perhaps honey is the only exception). The more processed a food is, the longer the shelf life, and the less nutritious it typically is. The longer the shelf life of the food we eat, the shorter our lives will be.

ACTION STEPS

The following dietary pattern promotes a healthy body and helps us maintain healthy eyesight:

- ○ Eat whole foods in their natural forms; avoid processed foods with a long shelf life whenever possible.

○ Eat nutrient-rich fat from sources like avocado and fish high in omega-3 fatty acids, such as salmon, sardine and mackerel, which are excellent for vision.

○ Eat more fresh fruits and vegetables, legumes, whole grains, nuts, and seeds. These foods are rich in antioxidants, phytochemicals, fiber, vitamins, and minerals that can prevent eye diseases.

○ Limit or eliminate refined carbohydrates, such as sugar, white flour, and vegetable oils that are refined in high temperature. These foods lack nutritional value and can lead to chronic inflammation.

○ Limit or eliminate highly processed meats such as deli meat, bacon, ham, sausage, and hot dogs.

○ Depending on your overall dietary pattern, you may want to consider supplementing with vitamins and minerals.

HABIT #5
Get Enough Sleep

D ID YOU KNOW THAT Tom Brady, one of the best NFL quarterbacks, goes to bed at 8:30 p.m. and gets up at 5:30 a.m.? Three-time NBA champion LeBron James reportedly needs 12 hours of sleep a day. Swiss tennis legend Roger Federer sleeps 10 to 12 hours each night to perform at his highest level. These peak performers know the importance of good shut-eye.

Sleep supports and aids our body and brain. It is an important factor for our general physical health and emotional well-being. We suffer health consequences if we don't get enough sleep. During sleep the brain grows and rewires itself, and releases hormones to repair cells. Dr. Matthew Walker, a neuroscientist and sleep expert who wrote *Why We Sleep, Unlocking the Power of Sleep and Dream,*[1] claims sleep and dreams are like miracle drugs:

"Sleep enhances our ability to learn, memorize, and make logical decision. It recalibrates our emotions, restocks our immune system, fine-tunes our metabolism and regulates our appetite. Dreams mollify painful memories and create a virtual reality space in which the brain melds past and present knowledge to inspire creativity. Sleep can

improve learning, mood and energy levels; regulate hormones; prevent cancer, Alzheimer's and diabetes; slow the effects of aging; increase longevity; enhance the education and lifespan of children; and boost our efficiency, success and productivity."

The visual system is an important brain function; thus, sleep affects vision. The article "Inverse Relationship between Sleep Duration and Myopia"[2] published in the peer-reviewed journal *Acta Ophthalmologica* links the association between sleep duration and myopia, according to a population-based, cross-sectional study of 3,625 Korean children aged 12–19 years. The researchers found that for every additional hour of sleep, the refractive error increased by 0.10 diopter. Remember, myopia is measured as negative diopters: this means the more sleep, the lesser degree of myopia.

Another study published in *Scientific Reports* (by the publisher of *Nature*) "Decreased Sleep Quality in High Myopia Children"[3] indicated that myopic children are late and short sleepers. For example, the high myopic children in the study went to bed approximately 74 minutes later than non-myopes and had one hour less sleep. The researchers suggested such sleep habit could affect systemic and ocular health if continued for several years, because sleep duration is closely related to health and growth in adolescence. As both myopia and sleep disorders are very common in children, they should be taught appropriate sleep behaviors both at home and in schools.

Sleep issues have become more common with the introduction of technology. Your tech habits can impact your sleep quality. According to National Sleep Foundation, using electronic devices before bedtime can be physiologically and psychologically stimulating in ways that can adversely affect your sleep. The more electronic devices that a person uses in the evening, the harder it is to fall asleep or stay asleep. *Chronobiology International*, a peer-reviewed journal published a study "Evening Light Exposure to Computer Screens Disrupts Human Sleep, Biological Rhythms, and Attention Abilities."[4] The researchers found that short-wavelength blue light, emitted by the screens we watch (computers, smartphones and tablets), damages the body's sleep-wake cycle, the duration of sleep, and even more so, the quality of our sleep. The blue light in the range of 450–500 nanometer (nm) wavelengths suppresses the production of melatonin, a hormone secreted at night that relates to normal body cycles and sleep. Screen light exposure in the evening may have detrimental effects on human health and performance. There are also indications that electromagnetic fields (EMF) from mobile phones and devices influence brain activity during sleep—don't leave them on in the bedroom.

Today, more and more people, including health professionals, believe the way to a more productive and more joyful life is getting enough sleep. Sleep is one of the cornerstones of health. We can regain control of our lives by developing a good sleep routine.

ACTION STEPS

○ Make sleep a priority! Get enough sleep to stay healthy, happy, creative, and smart!

○ Stick to a sleep schedule. Go to bed and wake up at the same time each day. To help you remember, set an alarm for bedtime, not just for wake up. Since we are creatures of habit, try not to have irregular sleep patterns across the week. Stick to a fixed schedule (that includes the weekend) for the optimal functioning of biological clocks and the quality of sleep.

○ Children and teenagers need eight to ten hours of high-quality sleep each night to function the best.

○ Don't eat, drink, or exercise within a few hours of your bedtime.

○ Make your room a sleep haven: keep it cool, quiet, and totally dark.

○ Stop using electronic devices (computer, tablet, or smart phone) two hours before bed if you can.

○ Keep your electronic devices off or out of the bedroom.

○ Read habit #20 on forming an effective evening routine.

HABIT #6
Mind Your Posture

THERE IS AN UNEXPECTED link between posture and eyesight. The eyes are part of the complex central nervous system, connected directly to the brain. Eyes accept light beams, which the rod and cone cells in the retina translate into electrical impulses. These impulses then travel on the optic nerve to the brain's visual cortex. In here, the brain interprets the signals and sends messages down the spinal cord to tell the rest of the body how to react to what the eyes see.

Good posture allows smooth communication between the eyes, the brain, and the spine. However, a slumped or hunched posture affects the connection quality between the spinal cord and the brain. People who have poor eyesight may squint, lean forward, slouch, or tilt their heads into an unnatural position to see more clearly. These movements create muscle tightness in the shoulders, neck, and head. Over time, this maladjustment can decrease the impulse connection with the eyes. According to the Cambridge Institute for Better Vision, nearsighted people often hold tension in their upper back, shoulders, base of the neck, and around the eyes. This tension continues even while sleeping, affecting pulmonary function and limiting the free movement and functioning of the eyes.

The AOA's *Clinical Practice Guideline. Care of the Patient with Myopia*[1] recommends this visual hygiene in vision therapy: read or do other visual work using a relaxed upright posture. A good posture ought to feel comfortable, natural, and energizing, not stiff or tiring.

In the 2016 study "Associations of Reading Posture, Gaze Angle and Reading Distance with Myopia and Myopic Progression,"[2] the researchers pointed out that the highest myopia progression is from the group who "read sitting down at baseline"; the lowest, from the group who "read faceup lying down." Reading with eyes turned more downwards was slightly connected with greater myopic progression.

In the study "Influence of Near Tasks on Posture in Myopic Chinese Schoolchildren,"[3] the researchers observed close working distances among these children. They found that near working distance and head declination can be affected by the attention dedicated to each task, the task difficulty, and the page/screen size. For example, handheld video games were associated with the closest working distance and head declination, which can lead to myopia progression, as shown in several other studies.

Dr. William Bates, the pioneer of healing vision naturally, once wrote in the *Better Eyesight Magazine* about balanced posture relating to eye diseases such as high nearsightedness, night blindness, and retinitis pigmentosa. He stated that a great posture balances the body—meaning whether or not it is at rest or in motion, its center of gravity is always kept exactly over its base. The spine is perfectly straight, the waist muscles firm, and the weight, in the standing posture, is supported upon the balls of the feet; in the sitting posture, is supported upon the thighs. He also discovered sleeping with a straight spine (i.e., sleeping on one's back with lower limbs completely extended and arms lying straight by the sides) to be very effective in improving the vision and relieving fatigue.

Silicon Valley's posture expert, Esther Gokhale, teaches similar postures, such as stretch-sitting, stack-sitting, and tall-standing. She points out that each muscle, bone, and ligament have its natural place. The design of the human skeleton, the end product of millennia of collaboration between gravity and structure, has a natural balance and harmony. When we restore that balance, the result is stillness and flow.

Several natural vision coaches reveal that when their clients reclaim their vision, they usually have much better posture as a side benefit. Or perhaps their posture provides a positive feedback loop in improving their vision. Endmyopia.com, a website created by Jake Steiner, a myopia reversal advocate, cited positive changes in the posture of his students who had showed promising improvement of their eyesight.

Good posture has many additional benefits: increased lung capacity, improved circulation and digestion, increased self-confidence, and increased energy levels. The Harvard Business School social psychologist, Amy Cuddy, and her research team studied the impact of high-power poses through the study "Power Posing: Brief Nonverbal Displays Affect Neuroendocrine Levels and Risk Tolerance."[5] The researchers were stunned by the impact that body language had on hormones within the body. They discovered several simple high-power poses increased testosterone (increased feelings of confidence) by 20 percent, and decreased cortisol levels (less stress) by 25 percent—in just two minutes! These power poses are *expansive* poses by taking up more space, and *open* poses by keeping limbs open. Both forms enhance presence and confidence. I encourage you to watch Cuddy's famous TED talk "Your Body Language May Shape Who You Are."[6]

Making great posture a habit requires awareness and practice. The good news is when you become mindful of all the tightness and tension, both you and your muscles will be very glad to let go. A proper posture goes a long way towards promoting better vision, physical health, and emotional health.

ACTION STEPS

To help you correct your posture, I suggest you use a mirror until it becomes second nature. Or you can enroll in courses taught by posture teachers such as Esther Gokhale.

Brian Johnson, a wise entrepreneur and the creator of *Philosopher's Notes*, once wrote a note called "Head threads, Power pose, and Thor's hammer." I found it to be one of the best posture instructions.

1. Head threads: Imagine having a thread that runs from the top of your head down through your spine. Gently pull it up—lengthening (and widening) your spine. When you sit. When you stand. When you walk. All day, every day. It's one of the keys to grace and poise.

2. Power poses: Channel your inner Superman or Wonder Woman. When you sit. When you stand. When you walk. Choose open and expansive power poses. All day, every day. It is one of the most effective ways to cultivate your presence and power.

3. Thor's hammer: Chest up. Chin down. All day. Every day. Thor's actor, Chris Hemsworth, confirms that it does a body good.

HABIT #7
Practice 20-20-20

OTH THE AOA (AMERICAN Optometric Association) and the AAO (American Academy of Ophthalmology) recommend the rule of 20-20-20 as a way to reduce eye strain[1]. The rule says that for every 20 minutes spent in near work (looking at a screen, reading, or writing), a person should look at something in the distance (20 feet or more away) for 20 seconds. Long periods of near work cause the muscles around the eyes strain and looking into the distance relaxes them. The 20-20-20 rule is one of the most obvious, effective, and easy-to-implement ways to prevent eye strain— just take frequent breaks. But even as the writer who promotes the rule, I did not do it well until now. In the action steps below, I share with you a couple of useful methods.

According to the global research company Nielsen, American adults spend over 11 hours per day listening to, watching, reading, or generally interacting with media in 2018.[2] The Vision Council reports that 70 percent of American adults report their child(ren) receives more than two hours of screen time per day. These children experience headaches, neck and shoulder pain, eye strain, dry or irritated eyes, reduced attention span, poor behavior, and irritability.[3]

The 20-20-20 rule was first coined by Dr. Jeffery Anshel, an optometrist and corporate vision consultant in California in the early 1990s. Dr. Anshel lectured in the corporate world on relieving computer vision stress, which leads to myopia and late-day headaches in a person's late 30s. He recommended visual ergonomics in the workplace that include the 3B rule—blink, breathe, and break, and the 20-20-20 rule for the break.[4]

The article "Computer Vision Syndrome: A Study of Knowledge and Practices in University Students"[5] explains why the 20-20-20 rule works. The researchers examined the eye symptoms as a result of prolonged working on a computer in 795 university students. They found that those who periodically refocused on distant objects while using the computer had fewer symptoms of computer vision syndrome, which includes eye strain, watering or dry eyes, headaches, and blurred vision. The dryness of the eye is caused when people forget to blink their eyes often while using a computer. It can be relieved by blinking very slowly for 10 times to rewet the eyes every 20 minutes. The headaches and blurred vision are caused by eye strain, which can be relieved by looking in the distance and taking deep breaths.

Dr. William Bates noticed while people with poor vision stare and strain to see everything at once, people with perfect sight shift their point of focus many times every minute, all day long. All that shifting sounds like a lot of work, but brain science tells us that our minds need a constant supply of new information to stay activated, interested, and relaxed. It also helps expand the brain's attention span. Taking regular breaks during near work with the 20-20-20 method not only prevents eye strain, but also keeps our brain stimulated in a natural way.

ACTION STEPS

○ Follow the 20-20-20 rule for visual hygiene. Set an alarm for every 20 minutes so you can look at the distance and relax your eyes. For the alarm, download a free app such as EyeCare, or use a pomodoro timer to remind yourself to take breaks.

○ Adopt computer eye ergonomic practices like the following from *The Program for Better Vision*:[6]

❑ Sit as far as possible, at least 25 inches, or an arm's length, from the computer screen.

❑ Position the screen so your eye gaze is slightly downward to the center of the screen. Use an upright, relaxed posture.

❑ Use anti-glare screens or eliminate the glare on the screen.

❑ Light the room appropriately. Lighting should not cause glare; use overhead, background, and foreground lighting that are not distracting.

❑ Blink every three to five seconds. Blink slowly 10 times every 20 minutes.

❑ Follow the 20-20-20 rule to reduce fatigue.

❑ Take frequent mini breaks to stand up, stretch, and move your body.

❑ Consider computer glasses if appropriate.

❑ See more than the screen. Being more aware of your surroundings and peripheral vision can reduce visual stress and fatigue.

HABIT #8
Do Your Eye Exercises

E XERCISE IN GENERAL IS a great investment in our health and wellness. Dr. Robert Lustig, one of the World's leading endocrinologists, talks about consistent exercise as a form of medicine in his book *Fat Chance:*[1] "Irrespective of weight, consistent exercise (even just fifteen minutes a day) is the single best way for people to improve their health. That is 273 hours paid in for 3 years of life gained, or a 64,000 percent return on investment. The best deal of medicine." While aerobic activities increase the circulation and oxygen supply to the upper body, including the brain and eyes, any form of deliberate exercise does your body good. When the body is healthy, the eye is healthy. But this book only focuses on eye exercises for myopia prevention and reversal.

Traditional Chinese acupoints massage

The elementary school I attended in China required mandatory eye exercises every morning. The school broadcasted instructions with music through the intercom, and all students performed acupoint self-massage for five to ten minutes. Although I had no hard proof of its effectiveness, almost all my classmates were able to maintain good eyesight until middle school when the routine stopped.

In a 2013 published study "Eye exercises of Acupoints: Their Impact on Refractive Error and Visual Symptoms in Chinese Urban Children,"[2] the researchers found the traditional Chinese eye exercises of acupoints appeared to have a modest effect on relieving near vision symptoms among Chinese urban children aged 6 to 17 years. But no remarkable effect on reducing myopia was observed. However, the researchers found a "seriousness of attitude" towards performing the eye exercises of acupoints showed a protective effect towards myopia. They pointed out that attitude, speed of exercise, and acquaintance with acupoints were all significant.

Another study called "Eye Exercises Enhance Accuracy and Letter Recognition, but Not Reaction Time, in a Modified Rapid Serial Visual Presentation Task"[3] suggests that eye exercises may prove useful in enhancing cognitive performance on tasks related to attention and memory over a very brief course of training.

Eye exercise has been criticized by many due to the absence of scientific research that demonstrates they can effectively reduce or eliminate refractive errors and decrease the need for corrective lenses. Even in China where eye exercise originated, the study "Chinese Eye Exercises and Myopia Development in School Age Children: A Nested Case-control Study"[4] showed no association between eye exercises and the risk of myopia onset or myopia progression. The group who performed high-quality exercises had a slightly lower myopia progression of 0.15 D than the children who did not perform the exercise over a period of two years.

However, while it is true that studies on the efficacy of eye exercises are lacking, researchers agree it is partly due to the absence of simple assessment tools in doctors' offices. Despite the arguments, Chinese acupoint eye exercises with a sincere attitude can be very beneficial to our eyes—just the simple fact that we are slowing down and giving our eyes undivided attention and tender/loving/care (TLC) can do wonders. Even though the exercises (described in the action steps) look too simple to improve your vision right away, the upside potential is still big. I came across many anecdotal success stories during my research for this book, in addition to my brother-in-law and my son's testimonials.

The Bates method

Most natural vision improvement and myopia reversal coaches in the US and Europe find their roots in the Bates method. The renowned ophthalmologist Dr. William Bates introduced the concept for improving eyesight in his book *The Bates Method for Better Eyesight Without Glasses.*[5] In his effort to restore natural habits of seeing, which are lost through strain, tension, and misuse of the eyes, Bates presented relaxation exercises to help the eyes and mind work together effectively.

Dr. Anshel, the optometrist who coined the 20-20-20 rule, regularly performed eye exercise techniques that helped him avoid using reading glasses (farsightedness) until age 50. He claims the techniques work muscles inside the eye, keeping the lens flexible and more able to adjust to different focal lengths.

Martin Sussman's *Program for Better Vision* is a modern program with a root in the Bates method. It has been around for decades helping numerous people regain their vision. It is perhaps the most comprehensive program I have seen—including two stages, close to 30 exercises, and several meditations. However, it was a little complicated for my then ten-year-old to stick with the schedule and exercises. But if you are a disciplined person, I strongly recommend you seek out that program.

None of the variations of eye exercises are difficult. But it is hard to stay with all of them on a regular basis. I suggest you try all the exercises listed in the action steps, then choose the ones that you like, and do them daily for at least 66 days. According to a study by University College London, 66 days is the average magic number to form a new habit like second nature, such as washing your hands after using the toilet.[6]

As said by Dr. Christiane Northrup, a visionary health expert, author, and speaker, "Our eyes respond to our thoughts and beliefs. When we believe the eye exercises are good for us, improvement happens. I personally found the palming and Chinese acupressure work the best for me. I love palming, and thumb-horizon (near-far) exercises the best." Palming, sunning, looking at nature, and the Chinese acupoint massage are my favorites—I found them calming, soothing and relaxing. Now it is your turn to find out your best exercises.

ACTION STEPS

The following exercises are not an exhaustive list, many natural vision improvement coaches have their own sets of exercises. Feel free to add them to your routine if you feel they relax your eyes, mind and body.

- ○ Palming for total relaxation. Rub the palms of your hands vigorously until they are warm. Close your eyes and place your palms gently over your eyelids, breathing slowly and deeply into your belly. Let the warmth of the palms transfer onto the eyes. You can feel the eye muscles relax as your eyes find relief in the darkness. Persist until the heat from the hands has been completely absorbed by the eyes. Repeat two to three times, or a total of five minutes.

- ○ Sunning. Keep your eyes closed while facing the sun and breathing slowly, then gently turn your head from side to side and from shoulder to shoulder for 15–20 times. Follow it with the above palming exercise for about 8–10 breaths.

Repeat two more times. The total time should be around five minutes.

I recommend you start this exercise at sunrise or sunset. Don't wear prescription glasses, contact lens, or sunglasses. Surrendering to the sun briefly each day can make a huge difference in terms of your vision and your overall feeling of well-being. It increases the eyes' sensitivity to light by stimulating the rods and cones of the retina which are responsible for light perception.

○ Improving color perception by stimulating cone cells. With eyes closed, look in the direction of the sun or a full spectrum of light for 15 to 20 seconds. With eyes still closed, gently massage the eyeballs with the fingertips for another 15 to 20 seconds. Continuing to keep your eyes closed, gently turn your head away from the sun and back until the whole range of the color spectrum is exposed.

○ Looking into the distance. This can be a part of the 20-20-20 routine. In this exercise, you look at the sky, the clouds, the hills, the valleys, the ocean waves, the night sky, or simply look out your window at trees. Don't "try" to see, as this will strain your eyes. Instead, simply notice what you can or cannot see. This helps prevent or decrease rigidity in the lens, and improves their flexibility, pliability, and elasticity.

○ Focusing (near-far exercise). Start by looking at an object up close and then at a distance. You can also do this by stretching your arm and lifting your thumb, first look at your thumb, then look into the distance as far away as you can, such as the horizon. Repeat this exercise for 15 times without straining. This exercise changes the focal length of the lens and improves the internal muscles of the eyeballs.

○ Distant reading. Pin up on the wall some reading matter, such as a Snellen chart. Every day move back a little bit to read it.

○ Hydrotherapy. Dip a washcloth in warm water and hold it against your closed eyes for 30 seconds. Repeat using a washcloth dipped in cold water. Repeat warm-cold-warm-cold for several minutes.

○ Blinking. Sit comfortably with your eyes open. Blink 10–15 times very quickly. Close your eyes and relax for 20 seconds. Repeat these five times.

○ Performing Chinese acupoint self-massage with a sincere attitude.

  ❏ Wash your hands. Sit down in a relaxed position, close your eyes, relax your shoulders and neck muscles, relax your facial muscles, and take several deep abdominal breaths.

❑ Massage each of the following acupoints for about 30 seconds:

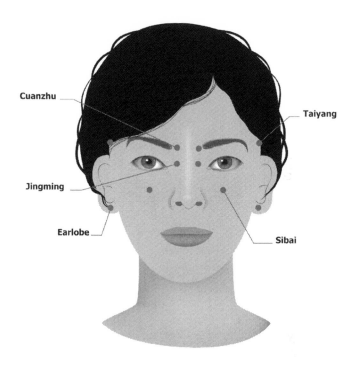

Figure 3   *Acupoints*

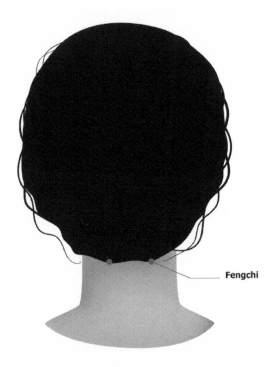

Figure 4 *Acupoints*

❑ Massage the "Cuanzhu" acupoint. It is
located on the inner tip of the eyebrow
where the bridge of the nose and eye socket
meet. Press and massage both sides with
your thumbs, with the other fingers relaxed
and gently placed on your forehead.

❑ Massage the "Jingming" acupoint. It is
located between the inner corner of the
eyes and the nose. Massage both sides in

an up-and-down motion with your index fingers.

❑ Massage the "Taiyang" acupoint. Place your index fingers or middle fingers on the hollowest parts of both sides of your temples—the "Taiyang" acupoint. Start massaging in a circular motion either clockwise or counterclockwise. Alternate directions halfway through the exercise.

❑ Massage around the eye sockets. The skin around your eyes is very thin, so use your ring fingers to apply the least amount of pressure. Gently massage the upper and lower bony parts of your eye sockets.

❑ Massage the "Sibai" acupoint. Look straight ahead and smile! While you're smiling, draw a straight line upwards from the corner of your mouth towards the pupil, and stop in the middle (between the pupil and the corner of your mouth). Gently press your index fingers into your cheeks on both sides and massage in a circular motion.

❑ Massage the "Fengchi" acupoint. Fengchi is where your skull meets the neck at the two hollow parts located on the back of your neck, a little below the level of your ears. Close your eyes. Use both index fingers and middle fingers to gently massage them in a circular motion. This is an excellent relaxation technique during stressful times.

❑ Massage the earlobes. Use the thumbs and index fingers of both hands to massage the center of each earlobe. Meanwhile, move all toes on both feet back and forth rhythmically (catch-earth movement) without moving the feet.

❑ Finally, do a quick palming session and imagine your eye muscles are fully relaxed.

○ Eye movements. The following exercises are recommended by Deepak Chopra, a medical doctor, and world-renowned pioneer in integrative medicine and personal transformation. The exercises strengthen the external muscles of the eyeball which are responsible for eye movement and coordination. Start with holding your head up, looking straight ahead. Hold each of the following positions for 15 seconds.

❑ Look up and to the left. This movement strengthens the ability of visual recall.

❑ Look down and to the left. This movement accesses auditory memory and the recall of a musical tune.

❑ Look up and to the right. This movement accesses the ability to create new visual forms.

❏ Look down and to the right. This movement accesses kinesthetic recall such as an experience of touch.

❏ Look directly to the right. This movement accesses the ability to create new sound forms.

❏ Look down to the end of your nose. This movement accesses the ability to strengthen olfactory sense.

❏ Look down toward your tongue. This movement accesses the ability to strengthen gustatory senses.

❏ Look upward and inward trying to look at the space between the eyebrows. This movement accesses the ability to heighten intuition.

Do all the exercises on both eyes without glasses or contact lenses. In order to get the benefits, choose your favorite exercises and do them daily with a sincere attitude. Rest for 10 seconds between exercises by closing your eyes.

Don't over exercise or it will cause strain or fatigue, and if you have any health concerns, you may need to avoid some or all of the exercises.

HABIT #9

Limit Your Use of Prescription Lenses

D<small>R. WILLIAM BATES CLAIMED</small> that the need for eyeglasses can be reversed by relaxation. Today, many vision coaches suggest minimizing the time you wear prescription lenses if you want to reach quantifiable vision improvement, because prescription glasses for myopia may lead to accelerated progression.

Eyeglasses

Eyeglasses are the most common form of eyewear used to correct myopia. The glasses use concave lenses, which are thinnest in the center. The numerical prescription in diopters is always marked with a minus (-) symbol.

Although your doctor may say you are free to wear glasses all the time, I recommend you limit their use to two to three hours a day if possible, and only wear them for distance vision. Children who wear glasses for close-up work may develop lens-induced myopia. When I worked in the ophthalmology devices industry for several years, I observed that the eye doctors always took off their glasses when doing near work.

As explained in habit #2, you can ask your doctor to give you an under-corrected prescription. This will give you 20/40 visual acuity instead of full 20/20 clarity. It will allow you to see well enough for most activities but leave room for your own natural vision to improve through the practices listed in this book. Keep looking for situations to use your natural vision and accept the blur with a peace of mind. The key rule is to never strain or squint when you are not wearing glasses.

Contact lenses

Contact lenses are worn directly on the cornea of the eye to correct refractive errors. They are considered medical devices and are regulated by the US Food and Drug Administration (FDA).

For children who are active in sports, contact lenses offer obvious advantages over glasses, such as safety and convenience. Some myopic children also think their self-esteem and self-confidence are enhanced with contact lenses. According to the study "Benefits of Contact Lens Wear for Children and Teens,"[1] more than 70 percent out of the 169 children and teenagers in the study prefer wearing contact lenses to wearing eyeglasses.

However, contact lenses have many disadvantages too. According to the study "Contact Lens-related Complications: A Review,"[2] many contact lens wearers experience complications from discomfort and infections, to edema and lesions. The longer one wears contact lenses, the greater the risk. The FDA also warns that wearing contact lenses puts you at risk of several serious conditions including eye infections and corneal ulcers. These conditions can develop very quickly and can be very serious. In rare cases, these conditions can also cause blindness.[3]

Another drawback is that you must do your near work with distance vision contact lenses. The lenses change your eye's focal plane and may cause lens-induced myopia with worsening vision.[4] Thus, you must reduce the time you wear contact lenses to a minimum, such as in sports and performances. Never wear them for too long, and definitely do not fall asleep with the lenses on. Remember, your cornea needs oxygen, and your eyes need a break from the lenses.

The general rule is to always look for ways to reduce the amount of time that you use your prescription lenses. Find opportunities to use your natural vision as much as possible. If you must wear them for long periods of time, then consider using under-corrected lenses.

Finally, I encourage you to develop a positive mental attitude—accept the status of your vision, do not fight for it, do not squint or strain, and do not compare it with others or what you should see. Make peace with your blur, form new habits listed in this book, and do something good for your eyes every day.

ACTION STEPS

○ Limit the use of your prescription glasses to two to three hours a day. Don't wear them for near work, such as reading, writing, and using computers/electronic devices. Only wear them when you need distance vision, such as driving, seeing a blackboard or white board far away, or going to a movie. Get an eyewear neck cord so you won't lose your glasses while constantly taking them off and putting them on.

○ Only use contact lenses in sports, onstage performances, or other occasions when eyeglasses are inconvenient.

○ Under-correct your prescription lenses if you plan to wear them daily.

○ Spend two to three hours a day outside without any prescription glasses. Give your eyes a break and room to breathe. Natural, unfiltered sunlight is vital for your eye health.

PART III: Mind

"There is no illness of the body
apart from the mind."

~ Socrates ~

"It's not the eyeballs fault when it changes its
prescription—it's the programming behind the eyeball.
It is what our brain is saying to our eyes to adapt
to the situation we're going through."

~ Dr. Sam Berne ~

HABIT #10
Reduce Your Stress Level

STRESS COMES WITH AN alarming statistic. According to the National Institute of Mental Health, 40 million adults in the US are affected by anxiety, and millions more are afflicted with depression-related disorders. The American Psychological Association's (APA) "Stress in America Survey" found that 30 percent of teens reported feeling sad or depressed due to stress, and 31 percent felt overwhelmed. The pressures of schoolwork, family life, social life, sports or other activities, combined with a relentless media culture, result in young people being more stressed than ever before. On average, teens report stress levels at 5.8 on a 10-point scale, compared with 5.1 for adults. Another poll by the social network After School found 45 percent of teens feel stressed all the time, based on a survey of 35,878 teenagers throughout the US.

Stress—coming from our environment, our body, and our thoughts—is key for our survival and a healthy dose of stress is a normal part of life. For example, we need stress in the form of "vertical vector" on our bones to keep them strong. We also need stress on our brains in order to learn new things. Many of us experience feelings of stress in the form of overwhelmingness, busyness, and tension from time to time, and then we recover.

However, chronic, unrelenting stress can be detrimental to our health: it weakens the immune system and promotes all kinds of diseases. When we are stressed, our bodies instinctively go into a "fight or flight" mode—because our body cannot distinguish between a life threat by a predator animal and modern-day stresses such as work pressures, family problems, or traffic jams. All stress triggers a cascade of hormones such as adrenaline and cortisol which speed up our heart rate, blood pressure, blood sugar, and blood flows to the limbs, all while enhancing coagulation (blood clotting in case of being bitten). It creates disharmony in our body, which physiologically expresses as lack of ease, or dis-ease.

The data from the study "Psychological Stress in Childhood and Myopia Development"[1] suggest that myopic children have more childhood stress based on retrospective childhood evaluations. There is no difference in experience of specific childhood stressors between the myopic and nonmyopic children. The data suggest, therefore, that myopic children may have perceptual problems related to recognition and interpretation of stressful situations in their lives. The researchers suggested that their findings point to possible unexplored risk factors for myopia, and complex interrelationships exists among psychological stress, childhood emotions, and myopia development.

In the study "Acute Psychosocial Stress Induces a Myopic Shift in Undergraduate Students / Conclusions,"[2] the researchers investigated the impact of near work and a stressful lifestyle on myopia. They found that a psychosocially stressful event contributed to an acute myopic shift in refraction in young adults undertaking tertiary study. These results suggest that acute psychological stress may play a role in driving environmentally derived refractive errors (myopia).

Even though our modern life is filled with stressors, we can interpret whether a situation is stressful or something we can handle with a little bit more peace. Stress only exists in the mind. Our thoughts, not the world, cause our stress. When we change our thoughts of the world, the world changes.

The study "Third-Person Self-Talk Facilitates Emotion Regulation without Engaging Cognitive Control: Converging evidence from ERP and fMRI"[3] published in *Nature's Scientific Report* reveals a simple solution for stress relief. Using one's own name during self-talk and moments of introspection rather than the first-person pronoun "I" increases peoples' ability to control their thoughts, feelings, and behaviors under stress. For example, say I, Aileen, am stressed out; instead of saying, "Why am I distressed?" I can say "Why is Aileen distressed?" The brain instantly displays significantly less activity in the emotional brain centers or in the region reflecting on painful emotional experiences. Third-person self-talk creates a psychological distance between the mind and our personal experiences. Therefore, it diffuses the influence of controlling emotions.

In her famous TED talk named "How to Make Stress Your Friend,"[4] health psychologist and lecturer at Stanford University Kelly McGonigal points out that we can handle stress differently, and even harness the energy of stress to work for us in our daily lives. Even when we are stressful, if we believe the stress is good for us to get our body and mind prepared, then our body reacts differently to stress. We may feel the excitement and heartbeat, but our blood vessels are relaxed. We will not be prone to diseases. In addition, McGonigal mentioned that when we see stress as a positive, we can access an unsung mechanism for stress reduction: reaching out to others for social support.

We can also explore other coping mechanisms, such as exercise, therapy, gratitude, prayer, deep abdominal breathing, meditation, tapping, yoga, or tai chi. For example, the study of meditators showed hospitalization rates decreased by 87 percent for heart disease; 55 percent for tumors; 30 percent for infectious diseases; and 50 percent for outpatient doctor visits.[5] Tapping, also called emotional freedom technique (EFT), has proven to reduce cortisol levels and improve psychological distress.[6] You can apply one or a combination of these tools so you can regain peace. When you are at peace, you are more creative in finding solutions to solve a problem or a challenge you are facing.

ACTION STEPS

○ Use third-person self-talk as a relatively effortless form of self-control in a stressful situation.

○ Choose to believe the stress is good for you in order to get your body and mind prepared. Then, you can deal with the stress more effectively without emotional triggers.

○ Use techniques to counter modern-day, low-level chronic stress: meditation, deep abdominal breathing, repetitive prayer, focusing on a soothing word (such as peace or calm), and visualization of tranquil scenes (such as a beach or green mountain).

○ Engage in physical exercises and other activities such as yoga, qi gong, tai chi and tapping.

○ Surround yourself with positive peer groups.

○ Reach out to others as the right social support enhances life experience.

○ Be aware that you are prone to having automatic negative thoughts. When feeling fear and doubts, replace them with questions like, "What if it all works out well?"

○ Reduce time spent on screens. Make time for idling, time for hobbies, or time in nature.

○ Get enough sleep (explained in habit #5).

HABIT #11

Manage Your Emotions

D
R. WILLIAM BATES BELIEVED vision problems are 90 percent mental and only 10 percent physical. Our past and present emotions can affect our vision. Strain and tension in the mind can cause unclear eyesight. Many vision coaches agree that myopia can be traced to some form of emotional strain, such as the suppression of emotions like fear, anger, sadness, or grief.

Martin Sussman discusses the link between emotion and eyes in his book *The Program for Better Vision*.[1] With his four decades of teaching natural vision improvement, Sussman points out that the underlying causes of not seeing clearly can often rest in the emotional and mental levels of vision. Through his programs, he observed that 70 to 80 percent of his students experienced a so-called "transitional period" (i.e., the time between seeing clearly with natural eyes and first noticing a limitation in physical vision [before glasses]). The transitional period is usually the year or so that precedes the visual limitation, when some major changes happened in a person's life in three areas: personal (such as puberty or aging), emotional (such as parents' divorce or a loved one dies), and situational (such as moving to another city or switching schools).

I have gathered many examples to prove this theory. My personal transitional period was the four months between when I was living at home and when I started boarding my high school at age 17. Within four months, my visual acuity deteriorated from 20/15 to 20/70. I first noticed my myopia symptoms when I saw halos around the moon. My son showed myopia symptoms eight months after his beloved grandparents moved to a different country. I also asked many myopic friends, most of whom can discover or acknowledge some form of emotional root to their vision problem. Population-based data also support the hypothesis that myopia was related with the presence of depressive symptoms among Chinese older adults.[2]

As cited in the previous chapter, the research "Psychological Stress in Childhood and Myopia Development"[3] studied more than 400 undergraduate students and asked them to evaluate their childhood stress. In the factor analysis, the myopia group had a significantly higher score on the stress-fear-abuse scale than the emmetropia (people with perfect vision) group. Psychological stress and childhood emotions are linked to children's myopia development.

Being nearsighted is an expression of how a person views and responds to the world. Nearsightedness is a way of seeing—or not seeing—that goes beyond seeing the eye chart's bottom line. When the outside changes happen in personal, situational, or emotional areas, they trigger our feelings and emotions. When we feel hurt or insecure, we don't want to admit to what we experienced, saw, or sensed. Coupled with strong emotions of fear and uncertainty, our mind develops a limited pattern of seeing. A part of us thinks if we pretend not to see it, it will disappear. This body and mind connection can turn our emotions into blurred eyesight.

Vision improvement involves transforming unresolved hurt. In Karol Truman's book *Feelings Buried Alive Never Die,*[4] the author encourages us to get in touch with our unresolved feelings. Those unresolved feelings during the transitional period that we pretend not to see can still be with us. They distort our happiness, health, well-being, and eyesight. We need to process these feelings, replacing the negative ones with a new, positive outlook. We have to give ourselves permission to feel sad, to mourn our losses, and to face unwanted change or failure. Then we can let go of the emotions through forgiveness and surrender, and be free to live fully in the moment of now.

In Sussman's book, he revealed that by recovering from early emotional decisions and healing painful memories, we can greatly accelerate vision improvement. The happy "side effects" are our inner peace and understanding, a clearer self-image, and a healthier attitude and perspective. Who wouldn't want to feel more serenity, love, joy, peace, and contentment?

Positive Emotion's Effect on the Eyes

Physiologically, all of our emotions and feelings are the result of chemical reactions taking place in our body. These reactions are responsible for making us feel negative emotions, like anger and sadness as well as positive emotions, like love and joy.

According to the study "Emotional States and Physical Health"[5] published in the journal of *American Psychologist*, positive emotional states may promote healthy perceptions, beliefs, and physical well-being. They help us build physical, psychological, and social resources, and motivate health-relevant behaviors. As anticipated by the Greek physician Hippocrates, positive emotions and healthy outcomes are linked through multiple pathways. For example, when we are happy, our body produces healthy doses of dopamine and nitric oxide. Research showed these neurotransmitters could slow eye elongation and prevent myopia.[6,7] Pleasant feelings also have direct positive effects on physiology, especially the immune system.

Now that we know negative emotions may lead to blurry eyesight and positive emotions prevent myopia, we can start forming new habits to tune ourselves to positive "channels" more often. I also encourage you to become an emotional archaeologist—to excavate buried feelings, partially forgotten hurts and unresolved issues that you did not want to look at. Only then can you shine your inner light upon them and set them free.

ACTION STEPS

○ See life as a great adventure. Be open to accept and embrace natural changes such as puberty and aging, or unpredictable changes such as illness and loss.

○ Use visualization to go back in time and resolve the buried feelings and hurtful emotions, such as failure, wounds, loss, fear, insecurity, misunderstanding, judgement, and other forms of emotional stress. Give yourself permission to feel sad and bad. Give each of these feelings a label. Acknowledge that you now have more tools and experiences to release them and move up to positivity. By processing these feelings, you can unlock these emotions, process them, shine your inner light on them, and transform them.

○ Cultivate positive qualities such as self-acceptance, self-compassion, and self-forgiveness. Give acceptance, compassion, and forgiveness to the "younger you" and others who caused you the hurt in the past.

○ Emotion is linked to stress; thus, how we handle stressful situations makes a huge difference. Remember to apply the methods to reduce stress outlined in habit #10.

HABIT #12

Relax Your Mind and Muscles Deeply

THE BODY IS ONE integrated system, not a collection of independent organs. The eyes, like the rest of the body, need proper rest and care. Your mental, emotional, and physical vision habits all play important roles in your vision health. A blurred vision reflects other imbalances in the body, mind, and spirit. Stress, force, pressure and tension, in addition to continuous close work can put strains on the eyes. These constant strains can take their toll. As we explained in habit #7 and #8, the eyes need rest every now and then, thus the 20-20-20 rule and eye exercises. In habit #10 and #11, we explained managing stress and releasing emotional strains. Here we focus on how physical relaxation can have a positive effect on the eyesight.

There are six muscles on the outside of the eye that move the eyeball. These muscles are small, but exceptionally fast and precise. They allow the eye to perform many complex tasks, like tracking moving objects, scanning for objects, and maintaining a stable image on the retina. Ideally, these muscles can easily move around and follow visual interests. The problem is that when these muscles strain and spasm, the vision starts to go; when they are relaxed, the vision remains clear.

In fact, just adding frequent breaks during a long near-work session has proven to be very effective to prevent myopia caused by near-work strain. The study "Nearwork-Induced Transient Myopia (NITM) Following Marked and Sustained, but Interrupted, Accommodation at Near"[1] found that by adding resting periods during a long and continuous near task, the participants avoided NITM. NITM has been reported to be additive after uninterrupted and sustained reading, but adding interruptions (rest periods) between each near task appears to prevent the cumulative effect (i.e., additivity effect).

As we discussed in earlier chapters, myopia starts out as a strain symptom—known as NITM or pseudomyopia. The AOA explains that blurred distance vision occurs when accommodation is not relaxed and advises that the goal of pseudomyopia treatment is relax-accommodation. Accommodation refers to the ability of the eye to change focus from near to far and vice versa. It is more effective to correct pseudomyopia through relaxation than prescription lenses. As we explained earlier, wearing lenses creates hyperopic defocus, which can be stimuli for the axial growth of the eye and cause progressive myopia.

Active mental relaxation

Vision goes deeper than the eyes and optic nerves, extending well into the layers of the mind, emotions, and spirit. According to *Psychology Today*, our minds carry our emotional stress, but our bodies do too. Research has proven that within the first few seconds of experiencing a negative emotion, people automatically tense the muscles in their jaw and around the eyes and mouth.[3] Multiple studies indicate that an increased mental workload results in increased muscle tension in the cervical and shoulder areas, particularly for people working at computers. These muscle tensions can decrease blood flow, lower oxygen delivery, and build up toxic metabolites.

To prevent storing negative emotions in our tense muscles, take a quiet moment to see where you might be storing stress in your body. By giving your body full attention and awareness, you can detect where you hold onto different emotions and kickstart the process of releasing them. When you maintain a relaxed state of mind, you can gain relaxed, natural vision. Some of the active mental relaxation tools are included in the action steps of the two previous chapters.

Atropine—chemical relaxation

It is worth mentioning the role of atropine in myopia control. You may be familiar with atropine—the dilating eye drops your doctor puts in your eyes during an eye exam. It helps open the pupils wide for close examination of the optic nerve and retina at the back of the eye. Atropine is all about eye-muscle relaxation. It causes the muscles in your eye to loosen up and widens (dilates) your pupil so that it will not respond to light.

Numerous studies find that atropine in extremely low concentration may prevent myopia onset as well as delay myopia progression in school-age children. In some Asian countries, it is considered one of the most effective therapies for myopia control.[4,5,6,7] The article published in *Nature* "Update In Myopia and Treatment Strategy of Atropine Use in Myopia Control"[8] reported recent clinical trials demonstrated low-dose atropine eye drops such as 0.01 percent resulted in retardation of myopia progression, with significantly less side effects compared to higher concentration forms.

When my son first had the myopic symptom, we used low-dose atropine over the weekend to relax his eye muscles. I believe it has contributed to his stable eyesight. Atropine has possible side effects, such as light sensitivity and near blur, so it must be administered by a professional. As a result, this method is not widely available and not practical for many.

The most practical ways to relax your eye muscles are included in habit #7 (practice 20-20-20) and #8 (eye exercises). Remember to relax them first thing in the morning, take frequent breaks during the day, and relax again before bed. The most practical way to relax your mind is through focused relaxation—by deliberately paying attention to thoughts and sensations without judgement. This allows the mind to refocus on the present moment. Remind yourself often to maintain a peaceful and relaxed state of mind as much as you can throughout the day.

ACTION STEPS

○ Reduce your mental stress and emotional strain by practicing habit #10 (reduce your stress level) and #11 (manage your emotions).

○ Reduce your physical strain by practicing habit #7 (20-20-20) and habit #8 (various forms of eye exercises).

○ Reduce time spent in near work if you can.

○ Add some outdoor time; blue skies and green nature always remind us to relax and stay calm and peaceful.

○ Accept and embrace your blur in a safe environment and do not strain.

PART IV: Environment

*The environment affects gene expression and phenotypes,
both in plants and animals.*

~ *Robert Feil & Mario F. Fraga* ~

EPIGENETICS AND THE ENVIRONMENT:
EMERGING PATTERNS AND IMPLICATIONS

*A rapidly growing body of research on populations in Asia
is yielding strong evidence linking diminishing levels of
exposure to outdoor light with a prevalence of myopia that
is approaching epidemic proportions.*

~ *Time Lougheed* ~

MYOPIA: THE EVIDENCE FOR ENVIRONMENTAL FACTORS.

HABIT #13
Go Outdoors and Play

TIME SPENT OUTDOORS IS perhaps one of the most explored topics in myopia research. Study after study, including cross-sectional, longitudinal, and interventional studies, shows that increasing time spent outdoors can protect people against myopia development. Researchers postulated that increased exposure to sunlight increases dopamine release in the retina, which reduces eye growth, and this hypothesis has been confirmed in a series of laboratory studies on experimental myopic animals.

Other studies pointed out that intense education and limited time outdoors play major causal roles in myopia epidemics.[1,2] Since outdoor light therapy presents little to no serious health concerns or side effects compared to other myopia treatments, it may be the ideal myopia treatment.[3] Encouraging children to play outside combats not only myopia, but also other major health concerns—childhood obesity, juvenile diabetes, and depression.[4]

In a Chinese study of 3,051 children aged 6–14 "Effect of Outdoor Activity on Myopia Onset and Progression in School-aged Children in Northeast China: The Sujiatun Eye Care Study,"[5] the researchers added two additional twenty-minute recesses outside the classroom in the intervention group of kids. The increased outdoor activities prevented myopia onset and development, as well as axial growth and elevated intraocular pressure (IOP) in these children.

The study "Near-Work and Outdoor Activities and the Prevalence of Myopia in Australian School Students Aged 12–13 Years: The Sydney Myopia Study,"[6] in which researchers included more than 2,000 randomly selected children from different ethnicities, concluded that outdoor activities were negatively associated with myopia (i.e., outdoor activities help prevent or reduce myopia). A similar study "Myopia Prevention and Outdoor Light Intensity in a School-based Cluster Randomized Trial"[7] also concluded schoolchildren with longer outdoor time in school (≥200 minutes) showed significantly less myopic shift. Among the 16 schools that were involved in this study, the outdoor promotion program effectively reduced the myopia change in both nonmyopic and myopic children. The researchers also observed that longer time in lower light intensity places, such as in hallways or under trees, is also an effective way to reduce myopia.

Another Sydney study "Outdoor Activity Reduces the Prevalence of Myopia in Children"[8] was published in *BMC Ophthalmology*. In this study, the researchers evaluated the effect of time spent outdoors on the development and progression of myopia among six-year-olds and 12-year-olds randomly selected from 51 Sydney schools. The 12-year-old children who spent more time outdoors had less myopia at the end of the two-year study period than others in the study—even after adjusting for the amount of reading performed, parental myopia and ethnicity. Children who performed the most amount of near work and spent the least amount of time outdoors had the highest mean amount of nearsightedness. Higher levels of total time spent outdoors, rather than just sport, were associated with less myopia.

The study "Myopia in Young Adults Is Inversely Related to an Objective Marker of Ocular Sun Exposure: The Western Australian Raine Cohort Study"[9] involved 1,344 of 19- to 22-year-old young adults. The researchers concluded the myopic refractive error was inversely associated with objectively measured ocular sun exposure, even after adjustment for potential confounders. This again supports the inverse association between outdoor activity and myopia.

The light-dopamine theory

Through the Sydney Myopia Study Group, Professor Ian Morgan and colleague Kathryn A. Rose, PhD, offer the light-dopamine theory—bright outdoor light stimulates the release of dopamine from the retina, and in turn, dopamine signals the sclera to inhibit axial growth. Dopamine is an important neurotransmitter in the retina and mediates diverse functions including (retina) development, visual signaling, and refractive development.[10]

The light-dopamine theory has attracted experimental support. In the laboratory, investigators have created experimental myopia in chickens[11] and nonhuman primates[12,13]. By simply increasing the intensity of light, the researchers were able to slow the myopia development in these animals. In another experiment using an animal model of myopia, researchers blocked the effects of dopamine with a dopamine antagonist, which also blocked its protective effect. A research conducted in Boston—where there's a big daylight variation—shows that myopia progression is three to four times faster in winter than in summer. In addition, the sunlight has 1,500 different wavelengths of light which all nourish the eye. Safe sun exposure is also the best way to optimize vitamin D levels, which support the function of muscle tissues around the lens of the eyes.

Outdoor time may bring many other benefits. Richard Louv, author and journalist, first coined the phrase Nature-Deficit Disorder in his bestselling book *Last Child in the Woods: Saving Our Children from Nature-Deficit Disorder*.[14] Nature-Deficit Disorder is the idea that human beings, especially children, are spending less time outdoors, and this change results in a wide range of problems such as obesity, negative moods, reduced attention span, and other behavioral disorders. We can safely add myopia as one of the problems. As Louv's research showed, direct exposure to nature is essential for healthy childhood development—physically, emotionally, and spiritually. It dramatically improves standardized test scores and grade point averages and develops skills in problem solving, critical thinking, and decision making. Even creativity is stimulated by childhood experiences in nature. In addition, nature is a potent therapy for depression, obesity, and ADD.

The environment provides an important health service. If you want to reduce your risk of developing myopia or reverse your existing myopia, you should spend more time outdoors under the sun without your smart phone or electronic devices. If you are a parent, encourage your child to go outdoors and enjoy playing sports, playing outside, and hiking. If you make decisions for a school system, you can change curriculum to include more outdoors time for children.[15,16]

ACTION STEPS

○ "Go outdoors and play" is a campaign by the Singapore's Health Promotion Board. Just do it!

○ Spend at least two–three hours outdoors or in the sun. Safe sun exposure is perhaps the best way to prevent or slow myopia progression.

○ Engage outdoor activities such as playing sports, hiking, biking, swimming, gardening, jumping rope, playing on the beach, or simply counting tree leaves.

○ Go out of your classroom during recess, look at the sky or trees. Rest your eyes.

HABIT #14
Control Indoor Lighting

W E ARE TURNING INTO an indoor generation. According to the Environmental Protection Agency (EPA), the average American spends 93 percent of our life indoors, which can be harmful to our health and well-being. Myopia is definitely one of the affected health areas. In the case of children, studies have shown that they spend only roughly one to two hours on weekdays in bright light (greater than 1000 lux, which is outdoor).[1-5] Thus, we spend most of our day in the general category of "less than bright" light exposure, mostly indoor light.

Research shows that children experiencing low average daily light exposure (342-576 lux) exhibited significantly greater eye growth (myopia) than children experiencing moderate (652-1019 lux) and high ($\geq$ 1020 lux) average daily light exposure levels.[5] The low average exposure refers to classrooms, homes, and study libraries—the places where children spend most of their indoor time. The study quoted in the previous chapter showed the children who were assigned to spend daily recess in a gymnasium—getting physical activity without outdoor light—were more likely to develop myopia over a one-year period than children who spent the same amount of time outside.

Animal studies have also proven this theory. A research showed that high illumination levels—comparable to those encountered outside—slowed the development of experimentally induced myopia in chicks by about 60 percent compared with normal indoor lighting conditions.[6] Researchers elsewhere have found similar effects in tree shrews and rhesus monkeys.[7-8]

In the "Pilot Study of a Novel Classroom Designed to Prevent Myopia by Increasing Children's Exposure to Outdoor Light,"[9] the researchers assessed light characteristics and user acceptability of a prototype Bright Classroom (BC) with an average 2,540 lux light intensity, designed to prevent children's myopia by exposing them to light conditions resembling the outdoors. Conditions were measured throughout the school year among the glass-constructed BC, a traditional classroom (with average of 477 lux), and outdoors (with 19,500 lux). Teachers and children both prefer and gave higher overall ratings to the BC. Ian Morgan, a professor at Australian National University and an authority in myopia research, talked about testing one alternative:

a specially engineered lamp that can create 10,000 lux, limited to the desk surface—to help prevent myopia.[10]

On the other hand, short exposure of extremely low light may be helpful for the eye. The research "Dim Light Exposure and Myopia in Children"[1] measured the amount of time children spent in scotopic (<1–1 lux), mesopic (1–30 lux), indoor photopic (>30–1000 lux), and outdoor photopic (>1,000 lux) light over both weekdays and weekends with wearable light sensors. The study found significant differences in average daily light exposure between myopic and nonmyopic children. During weekdays, myopic children spend significantly more time in mesopic light (dark indoors of 1-30 lux) than nonmyopic children; and on weekends, myopic children received significantly less scotopic light (<1-1 lux) and less outdoor photopic light (>1,000 lux) than nonmyopic children. In myopic children, the more time they spend in mesopic light (1-30 lux), the worse their myopic refractive errors. The researchers also observed that rod pathways are stimulated by dim light exposure (<1-1 lux, equivalent to darkness), which is good for the eyes. The conclusion? The optimal strategies for preventing myopia may include both darkness (scotopic light) and bright light (photopic light) exposure.

My brother-in-law Duncan used this strategy to its best—he counted tree leaves in the bright light and counted the stars in the night sky every day (in a relaxed way). He maintained his good eyesight till now, while I was the opposite. At age 17, I spent most of my time studying in classrooms with poor lighting along with no physical education or outdoor activities—the worst possible environment for my eye health.

Harmful blue light from screens and LED lighting

Although blue light from the sun can be good for our eyes, scientists have discovered that blue light, especially at shorter wavelengths, can damage cells in the retina, the light-sensitive layer of tissue that lines the inside of the eyes. For example, animal study results indicate that LED blue light exposure poses a great risk of retinal injury in awake, task-oriented rod-dominant animals.[11]

According to the Royal Society of Chemistry, blue light produces reactive oxygen species (ROS), such as superoxide radicals, in retinal cells. This can lead to cell death. ANSES (French Agency for Food, Environmental and Occupational Health & Safety) recently warns that the blue light in LED lighting that is increasingly used in our homes can damage the eye's retina while disturbing our biological and sleep rhythms. As discussed in habit #5, shortwave blue light suppresses melatonin, a hormone that regulates sleep–wake cycles. The study "Effect of Light Wavelength on Suppression and Phase Delay of the Melatonin Rhythm"[12] reveals the shorter wavelengths of 470, 497 and 525 nm (blue light) showed the greatest melatonin suppression, from 65 percent to 81 percent.

More and more studies are showing that the blue light from TVs, computer screens and smart phones can also damage human eye cells.[13] Experts suggest it is prudent to adjust screen brightness to be no brighter than needed to do the work or enjoy the entertainment.

ACTION STEPS

- ○ Increase the lighting in your home where you study or read, but try to avoid LED light if you can.

- ○ Consider reading or doing your homework outdoors in the shade. It is at least 1,000 lux even on the cloudiest day.

- ○ Dim light, such as the night sky, can be good for your eyes. Observe the stars for a couple of minutes before going to bed, don't strain your eyes. It is good relaxation.

- ○ Adjust the brightness of your TV screen and other electronic devices to be no brighter than needed to do the work or enjoy the entertainment.

- ○ Whenever you can, go outdoors and play!

HABIT #15
Remove the Night-light

T HE LINK BETWEEN NIGHT-LIGHT and myopia is controversial. However, I decided to keep this chapter, not only because of the possible link, but also because the night-light can disturb sleep cycles and inhibit the sleep-inducing hormone melatonin.

Children's eyes let in more light than adults' eyes do. The study "Myopia and Ambient Lighting at Night"[1] by researchers at the University of Pennsylvania revealed that night-lights are related to nearsightedness. About half the children (232) slept with a night-light, and 34 percent of this group became myopic. The smallest group was composed of the 75 children who slept in room light; subsequently, 55 percent became myopic. The overall myopia rate for the group was a shade under 29 percent. The researchers wrote, "The prevalence of myopia . . . during childhood was strongly associated with ambient light exposure during sleep at night in the first two years after birth."

However, the study "Myopia and Ambient Night-time Lighting"[2] by Ohio State University argues that leaving a light on in a sleeping infant's room won't increase the child's chance of becoming nearsighted, which contradicts the first study. Although the link between night-light and myopia was not firmly established, nighttime exposure to ambient light and various lighting displays were proposed as environmental hazards for sleep.[3-6] As we discussed in habit #5, sleep quality in children is significantly correlated with myopic error.

As parenting author Sarah Ockwell-Smith wrote in the *Huffington Post*, "Why Your Child's Night Light Is Ruining Their Sleep,"[7] night-lights, light shows, and glows from baby monitors have a devastating effect upon sleep because of the wavelength different colors of light have on the human body. White and blue based lights, however dim, will inhibit the secretion of melatonin at night. Melatonin is necessary for children to not only go to sleep initially, but also to stay asleep for longer overnight.

In his ground-breaking book *Why We Sleep*,[8] Dr. Matthew Walker cited the research he had led in the NICU (neonatal intensive care unit). In most NICUs, strong lighting often remains on throughout day and night, assaulting the thin eyelids of the infants who sleep most of the 24 hours. Dr. Walker's research team created dim-lighting conditions during the day and near-blackout conditions at night. In just a few months, his preliminary research findings from several NICUs showed that infant sleep stability, time, and quality all improved. Consequentially, they observed 50 to 60 percent improvement in neonate weight gain and significantly higher oxygen saturation levels in blood, relative to those preterm infants who did not have their sleep or environment prioritized. Amazingly, the well-slept preterm babies were also discharged from the hospitals five weeks earlier! According to the American Medical Association (AMA) journal, daily NICU costs exceed $3,500 per infant.[9] That is an estimated $73,500 USD in savings, on top of the long-term health benefits these babies gain. Again, tiny changes, remarkable results.

I like the slogan the *New York Times* writer Dr. Perri Klass created—"To Help Children Sleep, Go Dark."[9] I encourage you to create an ideal sleep environment by removing the night-lights, and all lights coming from electronic devices from the bedroom. Total darkness enhances sleep quality significantly. Create a peace haven for your precious sleep and regeneration time. If your child must sleep in a room with night-light for fear of darkness, then choose a dim reddish light to minimize disruptive effects on sleep cycles.

ACTION STEPS

○ Remove night-lights from all bedrooms. The best lighting is no lighting.

○ Tape over lights on baby monitors that are white, green, or blue. To help children sleep, go dark! If you have to keep a night-light, choose a dim red or orange hue lights for the child's bedroom.

○ Light all bathrooms with red or orange hue night-lights.

HABIT #16
Hang a Snellen Chart

D R. WILLIAM BATES FIRST introduced this practice for myopia prevention in the early 1900s. Dr. Bates discovered that our human eyes cannot see anything with perfect sight unless we have seen it before. When the eye looks at an unfamiliar object, it always strains more or less to see that object, producing an error of refraction. When children look at unfamiliar writing or figures on the blackboard or whiteboard, distant maps, diagrams, or pictures, the retinoscope always shows that they are myopic, though their vision under other circumstances may be absolutely normal. The same thing happens when adults look at unfamiliar distant objects. When their eye regards a familiar object, however, their vision is deemed normal. Not only can the familiar object be regarded without strain, but by first looking at a familiar object, the strain of looking later at unfamiliar objects is lessened. Dr. Bates discovered this while examining the eyes of 1,500 school children at Grand Forks, ND.[1]

In the early 1900s, at the request of the superintendent of the schools of Grand Forks, Mr. J. Nelson Kelly, Dr. Bates helped introduce a simple way to prevent myopia—the teachers hung an eye chart at the front of the classroom to act as the familiar object for all the students to look at whenever being introduced to new, unfamiliar objects. If the unfamiliar objects created blur, they could quickly glance over at the familiar eye chart to eliminate the blur. During the eight years of implementation, myopia among the children in Grand Forks reduced from six percent in the beginning to less than one percent at the end.[1]

A teacher of a class of 40 children in Grand Forks had kept a Snellen test card continually in her classroom. She directed the children to read it every day. For eight years none of the children under her care acquired defective eyesight. This method was later used in several public schools in New York City—over 1,000 children with defective sight restored to normal vision in both eyes. Dr. Bates published this study "Myopia Prevention by Teachers"[2] in 1913, now archived in the *American Journal of Ophthalmology*, Volumes 29–30.

Parents who wish to preserve and improve their children's eyesight can do the same. Just buy a Snellen test card at home and encourage the child to read it every day. This alone can help prevent myopia and other errors of refraction, and improve the vision even when it is normal. And if your child(ren) has imperfect vision, encourage them to read the card more frequently. Parents could also improve their own eyesight to normal so their children may not imitate wrong methods of using the eyes and will not be subject to the influence of an atmosphere of strain. But according to Dr. Bates, this practice will not help much while glasses are worn.

To use this method at home, hang the Snellen test card in an easy-to-access area. Read the card on the wall at a distance of 10, 14, or 20 feet and devote half a minute a day, or longer, to reading the smallest letters you can see with each eye separately, covering the other with the palm of the hand without touching the eyeball. Keep a record of the progress made. The records need to include the name and age of the person, the vision of each eye tested at 20 feet, and the date. For example:

- John Doe, 11, Aug 18, 2019
  - R. V. (vision of the right eye) 20/40
  - L. V. (vision of the left eye) 20/20
- John Doe, 12, Feb 18, 2020
  - R. V. 20/30
  - L. V. 20/15

The numerator of the fraction is the distance at which the letter is read, and the denominator is the distance at which it ought to be read. In the case of 20/40, the numerator 20 represents the person is standing 20 feet away from the chart, and the denominator represents a person with normal eyesight can read them 40 feet away. These numbers are posted next to their corresponding row of letters on the chart.

Based on Dr. Bates's research and experience, he was confident that children under 12 years who have not worn glasses are usually cured of defective eyesight by the above method in three months, six months, or a year![1]

ACTION STEPS

- ○ Go to Amazon.com and buy a Snellen Wall Eye Chart for about $10.

- ○ Hang the Snellen chart in an easy-to-access area. Read the chart on the wall at a distance of 10, 14, or 20 feet and devote half a minute a day, or longer, to reading the smallest letters you can see with each eye separately, covering the other with the palm of the hand without touching the eyeball. Keep a record of the progress made.

- ○ Other eye exercises with the Snellen test card:

  - ❑ Stand in such a distance where you can clearly see about half the chart.

  - ❑ Read the letters in each clearly visible row, letter by letter. Try to draw their contours and see them clear and black. During this exercise, blink frequently, close the eyes from time to time, and visualize the letter you have just read. Imagine that it is even blacker and sharper.

❑ When reading the chart, you can also raise your hands to the height of the eyes and move your fingers and palms. This will activate your peripheral perception and reduce the stress due to central vision.

❑ When you come to the row with non-recognizable letters, do not strain your sight. Try neither to see clearly nor to read them. Allow your eyes to move freely across the letters. Watch the space between the letters, noticing their blackness and shape. Take deep and slow breaths, blink, and wave your fingers. Once in a while, close your eyes and visualize the letters while repeating in your mind that the chart is white, and the letters are black.

❑ Move down the chart and when you reach its end, do a short palming exercise. Then, repeat the steps, but this time starting from the bottom of the chart. Watch if earlier visible contours of letters are now more visible. Accept what is blurred and enjoy every detail you can see clearly and without stress.

❑ Do this exercise as often as possible even if you have good vision—it helps maintain the good sight and even improve the sight to better than 20/20.

PART V: Habits

"We are what we repeatedly do.
Excellence, therefore is not an act, but a habit."

~Aristotle ~

"Your life today is essentially the sum of your habits.
How in shape or out of shape you are?
A result of your habits. How happy or unhappy you are?
A result of your habits. How successful or unsuccessful
you are? A result of your habits."

~ James Clear ~

HABIT #17
Make Vision Health Habitual

A HABIT IS A REDUNDANT set of automatic, unconscious thoughts, behaviors, and emotions that you acquire through repetition. It is when you've done something so many times, your body now knows better than your mind. The New York Times bestselling author Charles Duhigg, who wrote *The Power of Habit*,[1] claimed that the key to achieving success in any area of life—exercising regularly, losing weight, raising exceptional children, becoming more productive, building revolutionary companies and social movements—is understanding how habits work.

James Clear, author of *Atomic Habits: An Easy and Proven Way to Build Good Habits and Break Bad Ones*,[3] points out that changes that seem small and unimportant at first will compound into remarkable results if you're willing to stick with them for years. The tagline of Clear's instant New York Times bestseller is "tiny changes, remarkable results."

You might have heard the common myth that it takes 21 days of repetition to form a new habit. But the study "How Are Habits Formed: Modelling Habit Formation in the Real World"[2] published in the *European Journal of Social Psychology* investigated the process of habit-formation in everyday life. The researchers found it took on average 66 days to form a habit, such as eating a salad at lunch or exercising 30 minutes a day. In the study, the actual number of days ranged from 18 to 254 days—indicating that it can take a very short or a very long time.

Vision also has its habitual root. The Israel research article "The Influence of Study Habits on Myopia in Jewish Teenagers"[4] found a statistically significant higher prevalence and degree of myopia in a group of 193 Orthodox Jewish male students who differed from the rest in their study habits. The researchers found that Orthodox schooling is characterized by sustained near vision and frequent changes in accommodation due to the swaying habit during study and the variety of print sizes. This unique visual demand led to a possible myopic effect.[4]

Our eye care habitual routines are essential to our well-being. In our interaction with the environment, no other organ can compare with the contribution the eyes make. How we use our eyes and vision system dictates how well we survive in our environment. We cannot pass this responsibility to someone else, even doctors. We must take the full responsibility to form the habits to take good care of our eyes.

The study "Making Health Habitual: The Psychology of 'Habit-Formation' and General Practice"[5] revealed that patients trust health professionals as a source of advice on "lifestyle" (i.e., behavior) changes, even brief opportunistic advice can be effective. However, many health professionals shy away from giving advice on modifying behavior because they find traditional strategies for changing behavior time-consuming to explain, and difficult for the patient to implement. Furthermore, even when patients successfully initiate the recommended changes, the gains are often transient because few of the traditional behavior change strategies have built-in mechanisms for maintenance (i.e., few know how to form habits that last).

So how do you smoothly implement habit changes? The rule is to repeat a chosen behavior in the same context until it becomes automatic and effortless. James Clear suggests having a keystone habit—a behavior or routine that naturally pulls the rest of your life in line. Imagine how much easier and more fulfilling your life could be if you discovered one or two keystone habits that naturally put the rest of your day in place?

For Clear, his keystone habit is weightlifting. It triggers a wide range of secondary benefits, such as a getting a good workout, focusing better at work, eating better, sleeping better, and waking up the next day with more energy. For me, my keystone habit is a morning routine called SAVERS, which is discussed in habit #18. Even when I don't have time for the entire process, I still complete a short meditation and write down three small things I am truly grateful for. Doing this helps me wake up on the bright side and boost my sense of well-being. Another keystone habit is when I encounter a challenge or a difficulty, instead of internalizing it as a permanent failure, I repeat a saying I learned from Louise Hay: "All is well. Everything is working out for my highest good. Out of this situation only good will come. I am safe." It keeps me calm so I can think about solutions.

We cannot change our eyesight until we change something we do daily. Success is a long series of habits—small wins and tiny breakthroughs in each micro-moment. As James Clear puts it, "Every action you take is a vote for the type of person you wish to become. No single instance will transform your beliefs, but as the votes build up, so does the evidence of your new identity." So today, be committed to taking that first single step, and build your new identity as a person with perfect natural vision. Once you set your life to consistent rhythms as habits, you will feel the freedom.

ACTION STEPS

- ○ Decide on a goal that you want to accomplish. Write it down on the following table (adapted from the "*Making Health Habitual*" study[5]).

○ Choose a simple daily action that will get you closer towards your goal.

○ Plan when and where you will do your chosen action.

○ Every time you encounter that time and place, do the action.

○ Be consistent. It will get easier with time, and within 10 weeks, you could find you are doing it automatically without even having to think about it.

○ Congratulations, you've made a healthy habit that benefits your eyes!

My goal (e.g. Follow 20/20/20 rule as much as possible every day)

_____

_____

_____

_____

My plan (e.g. Use a pomodoro timer or an app on my phone. Stay focused for 20 minutes on a single task, then take a short break to look in the distance and relax my eyes)

_____

_____

_____

_____

(When and where) _____

I will _____

You can use a simple form to track your new habit until it becomes automatic. You can rate how automatic it feels at the end of each week on a scale of 1 to 10—1 being not automatic at all, 10 being completely automatic. Your confidence will grow as you watch it getting easier as time goes by.

New Habit Tracking Sheet								
Week	Mon	Tue	Wed	Thu	Fri	Sat	Sun	Rating (1-10)
1								
2								
3								
4								
5								
6								
7								
8								
9								
10								

HABIT #18
SAVERS Morning Routine

ROM PRESIDENTS TO CELEBRITIES, successful people credit their morning rituals as their key to success. If you read any personal development books, you will definitely come across the power of a morning routine. One phenomenon was started by an entrepreneur named Hal Elrod who wrote the book *The Miracle Morning*.[1] The book spread like wildfire, with many more miracle morning books published and dedicated to couples, parents, teenagers, college students, writers, entrepreneurs, salespeople, real estate agents, marketers, etc.

How we wake up each day and our morning routine (or lack of one) dramatically affects our productivity and success in every area of life. Do you wake up in a rushed, chaotic, stressful way? Or do you start your day in a calm, peaceful, and rejuvenating way? Now let's see how we can build a miracle morning routine that helps myopia prevention!

Hal Elrod's SAVERS morning routine (brief summary)

The SAVERS routine is borrowed from Elrod's *The Miracle Morning* book. I have been following this morning routine since I first read this book in 2015.

1. **S** is for silence. It refers to things such as meditation, prayer, deep breathing, and gratitude. The idea is to quiet your mind, block out the chatter, and start the day with calm thoughts.

2. **A** is for affirmation. Affirmations are encouraging words you tell yourself to achieve your goals, overcome fears, and be healthy and happy. Here, you take the full responsibility for actively choosing to think positive, proactive thoughts that will add value to your life.

3. **V** is for visualization. It is also known as creative visualization or mental rehearsal. It has long been a part of elite sports. High achievers such as Olympians, professional athletes, and business tycoons use visualization as mental training. Here, you can design the vision that will occupy your mind, ensuring that greatest pull on you in your future.

4. **E** is for exercise. Morning exercise has been the staple for many successful people. It significantly boosts your energy, enhances your health, improves self-confidence and emotional

well-being, and enables you to think and concentrate better. It can be an elaborated full-blown training routine or a simple five-minute aerobic exercise.

5. **R** is for reading. Reading is the fast track to transform any area of your life. It is one of the most immediate methods for acquiring the knowledge, ideas, and strategies to achieve a high level of success. The key is to learn from the experts and model their behavior.

6. **S** is for scribing (i.e., writing). A five-minute writing or journaling activity is a great way to process your thoughts and improve your mood. Journaling will also help you be more self-aware and more articulate. You can do it with a physical journal, a file on your computer, or an app, such as Five-Minute Journal, on a tablet or a phone.

Morning routine adapted for myopia prevention and eyesight improvement

Here is an example of morning routine for eye care. Of course, you can pick and choose the ones that fit your schedule and to your liking. Anything you enjoy doing will benefit your eyes and your body.

1. Silence. Sit down on a chair with your feet on the floor, spine straight, hands on your laps, and close your eyes. Take long and deep

breaths, feel grateful for your eyesight even though it may not be perfect. Let your eyes and your body relax, release all tension from your eyes, bless your eyesight, and imagine your vision becoming sharper and better. When you have random thoughts coming up, just acknowledge them, and then come back to focus on your breath and relaxing your eyes and your body. If you are new to meditation, start with a five-minute duration.

2. Affirmations. Stand tall, spine straight, and relax your shoulders with an elegant posture. You can also incorporate power poses, such as making a fist or hand gesture. Read your list of affirmation in a slow confident tone, generate authentic emotions, and infuse them into every affirmation and feel the truth. Say these affirmations or make your own adapted versions:

> I am grateful for my eyesight even if it is not as perfect as I wish it could be. My eyesight is naturally improving. I am releasing the tension around my eyes. My eyes are free from strain. I focus my eyes with ease. My eyes are becoming healthy and strong. I am healing my eyes. I can see clearly.[2]

3. Visualization. Sit up tall in a comfortable position, breathe deeply, close your eyes, and clear your mind. Start to visualize yourself living in your ideal day, seeing everything crystal clear, and performing all your tasks with ease, confidence, and enjoyment. To make the visualization more effective, you need to use all five senses—feel it, see it, smell it, hear it, taste it—as if you are living the life and the image you create in your mind. In this world, you can see everything perfectly. Do this for three to five minutes.

4. Exercise. If you don't have a morning exercise routine, do a five to ten-minute aerobic exercise, such as jumping jacks, burpees, or weightlifting, to get your blood and oxygen flowing to your brain and eyes. I suggest you do some simple eye exercises, such as palming, sunning, and acupoint massages outlined in habit #8.

5. Reading. Spend ten minutes reading an uplifting book. This will fill your brain with positive thoughts and ideas to improve yourself. Put all your favorite inspirational books in a special location on your bookshelf for easy access. If you read ten pages a day, you can amass roughly 18 books in a year.

6. Scribing. Do a five-minute dedicated journaling session. I love writing in a physical journal.

I think handwriting is an important tool in
the acquisition of reading and writing skills. I
always start by listing three new things I am
grateful for that day, then write down anything
that comes to my mind. They are usually in
the areas of experiences, accomplishment,
improvements, and challenges.

When all is done, remember to eat a nutritious whole
foods breakfast. Stay away from processed foods and
foods with added sugar. My favorite part of the breakfast
is a green smoothie. I often add a variety of green leafy
vegetables, berries and fruits, nuts and seeds, but no
sugar or artificial sweeteners. Smoothies are important
sources of fiber and antioxidants, and they are delicious
and energy boosting!

HABIT #19

PEACE Daily Routine

MOST WORLD EXPERTS HAVE powerful daily routines that serve as useful mental tools to create sustainable success. As Aristotle said, "We are what we repeatedly do. Excellence, therefore is not an act, but a habit." Let's look at how we can build our daily routine around myopia prevention and reversal.

PEACE daily routine

I have researched, implemented, and summarized the daily habits as PEACE for myopia prevention (acronyms anyone?).

1. **P** is for peace and presence. Having peace of mind despite life's chaos helps reduce our stress level. Presence is the state of being present, being aware of our own mental, emotional,

and behavioral patterns. It also means to bring mindfulness and attention into whatever we do. The following exercises help us cultivate peace and presence.

○ Take deep breaths frequently. A growing number of empirical studies[1] have revealed that diaphragmatic breathing may trigger body relaxation responses and benefit both physical and mental health. You can simply incorporate this into your daily life—whenever you can. Take slow and deep abdominal breaths (six to ten breaths per minute). I love box breathing, which has a calming effect on me: inhale to the slow count of four, hold your breath to the slow count of four, exhale to the slow count of four, then hold your breath again to the slow count of four. Repeat a couple of times.

○ Add a mini meditation in the afternoon when you feel your energy draining. Just close your eyes, breathe deeply, and tune into your body. Pay attention to your breath, and then different parts of your body. Relax your eyes and facial muscles, then relax each part of your body. You can also use meditation apps or YouTube videos for guided meditations if you prefer. Of course, other forms of stress reduction such as yoga, qi gong, and tai chi are also effective.

○ Remember to smile or simply fake a smile. A study published in *Psychological Science*[2] has shown that the mere act of smiling or faking a smile can lift your mood, lower stress, boost your immune system, and possibly even prolong your life.

2. **E** is for eye exercise. Incorporate these habits that promote eye health:

○ Practice 20/20/20—limit exposure of screens or other close work to 20 minutes at a time to avoid eye strain. Look into the distance at least 20 feet away for 20 seconds (habit #7).

○ Set aside time to practice eye exercises (habit #8), such as palming and Chinese acupuncture point massages.

○ Maintain a great posture all the time (habit #6).

○ Read an eye chart, especially when you are trying to see new information (habit #16).

○ Only use glasses (if you wear glasses) for distance vision. Take them off for near work (habit #9).

○ Never squint your eyes. Accept your refractive state as is; do not strain.

3. **A** is for active lifestyle. Schedule outdoor time and activities under the sun or in nature (habit #13). We are not designed to be sedentary beings. Our bodies are built to move. Children and adults who are in good aerobic shape are far less likely to experience myopia. Time in nature not only improves our eyesight, but also reduces stress and the risk of many chronic diseases.[3]

4. **C** is for concentration, which also means to focus on a single task. Concentration requires you to focus on the single most important task at a time until it is finished, then move on to your second most important task, and so on. World-class experts in nearly any field have one common characteristic: focus—as mastery requires focus and consistency.

   Most of us are inundated with work and tasks all the time. We rush and pride ourselves with the ability to multitask. Multitasking is not associated with being better; it only brings stress and distraction. Studies have shown that shifting between tasks creates brief mental blocks, and can cost as much as 40 percent of someone's productive time. We need to learn to slow down, focus on a single task that will move the needle, and let go of worries that we are out of control.

To apply this habit, I usually start planning my day the night before or in the early morning. I write down both a "to-do list" and a "not-to-do list," and prioritize the to-dos based on importance and urgency. Then I begin immediately on the most important task and focus on it until completion. Doing this alone, I can increase my productivity tremendously—just by planning, starting, and completing the most important tasks every day.

5. **E** is for eating a nutrition-rich diet centered on whole foods (habit #4). Each of us has a unique nutrition blueprint, so there is not a diet that fits all. However, most nutritional experts agree a healthy diet must have these components: fresh and non-processed foods, lots of fresh vegetables and fruits, high-quality protein and fat, nuts, seeds, legumes, and nutritional supplements if needed. These foods provide not only energy, but also the vital nutrients, fatty acids, fibers, antioxidants, phytochemicals, vitamins, and minerals that are essential for your eye health. Remove the foods that can cause inflammation—highly processed foods, refined sugar, and highly refined vegetable oils explained in habit #4.

HABIT #20

DREAM Evening Routine

A GREAT EVENING ROUTINE NOT only gives us a good night of sleep, but also lets us wake up with energy, clarity, and productivity. The more we maximize our evenings, the more we will find our following days fulfilled.

To establish that routine, we need to consider our mood. The mood we go to sleep in is often the mood we wake up in. Many people have the habit of reviewing all the things that did not work for them during the day, all the people who hurt their feelings, or all the worries they have about the future. Others watch depressing news or violent programs on TV. Then, they go to bed and marinate their minds in those negative thoughts for eight hours.

The empowered few have a different routine. They count their blessings and plant the seed of positive affirmations. As a middle-aged mom, I often battle a racing mind at bedtime. After studying some famous people's sleep routines, I have come up with the DREAM routine based on what worked the best for others and myself.

DREAM evening routine

1. **D** is for disconnect. Disconnect from the digital world two hours before bed—turn off big or small screens (TV, computer, tablet, and phones). Electronic devices put people in a reactive mode and bring stress. In addition, every hour of screen time postpones melatonin (the hormone that helps control our daily sleep–wake cycles) secretion by 30 minutes.

2. **R** is for reading. Reading a good paper book at night helps create an oasis of peace and serenity. Read a good fiction, a fun book, or an inspirational book. According to Dr. David Lewis, a cognitive neuropsychologist, "Losing yourself in a book is the ultimate relaxation." Don't read an e-book as we have just "disconnected" from all electronic devices in the previous step.

3. **E** is for eye exercises. The evening eye exercise can be simple; the key purpose is to fully relax the muscles around the eyes. One effective way is to look into the evening sky and count some of the visible bright stars. My favorite

relaxation is a five-minute palming exercise with deep breaths. You can also choose some exercises you like from habit #8.

4. **A** is for affirmations. The evening affirmations can be "I release today. I let go of any fear, anger, and blame. Instead of problems, I see solutions. I see the way things can work. I bless my experiences. I choose to regain my peace. I am grateful for all the things I have. I invite a good night of sleep. I see more clearly when I am relaxed and centered. Good sleep helps me regain crystal clear eyesight."[1]

5. **M** is for meditation. Meditating before bed can relax your nerves, calm your racing mind, and help you sleep better and deeper. Studies show that meditating before bed can cure insomnia and combat certain sleep disorders.[2]

   M is also for miscellaneous. I have benefited from the teachings by wise people like Leo Babauta from Zen Habits. He suggests writing down the three MITs (most important tasks) for the next day, checking the calendar, getting clothes ready, packing lunch, and tidying up so you are greeted with a clean house in the morning.

AFTERWORD

THANK YOU FOR READING this book. I sincerely hope that I provided some value in your journey to protect, honor, and care for your eyesight so it can function to its best. According to Dr. William Bates, perfect sight means perfect relaxation of the mind; it also means perfect memory and perfect imagination. When one is perfect—all is perfect. The opposite is also true.

Like you, I am also on this journey to restore my eyesight from decades of living with progressive myopia. I am very happy to report that my progression stopped several years ago, and I am recovering gradually. I am grateful for my son for bringing the message to me and letting both of us embark on this amazing journey to help us to regain our vision.

I know the habits seem simple and easy on paper, but I also know it is very difficult to build them into our daily routine. Believe me, I am at best practicing 50 percent of the things I am preaching, but they have made a huge difference in my life and my children's lives. Both my children were able to keep their vision well enough for daily academic and sports activities without glasses. I encourage you to re-read this book, pick up the habits that appeal to you, and implement them right away. Once you see some early successes, you will be excited and eager to add more lengthy exercises and habitual changes.

In my research, I have come across numerous case studies showing the great side effects of better vision—improved posture, improved confidence, letting go of tight neck and shoulders, headaches disappearing, etc. These new habits not only improve people's eyesight, but also expand their personal growth. Some even say the process is "to relearn to see and relearn to live." Let today be your day to start a new routine to nourish your eyesight. Appreciate all that you see now—and see to it that your good vision lasts a lifetime. I am very grateful for your trust, and I wish you the best in your journey.

BIBLIOGRAPHY

Introduction

1. Francisco, Bosch-Morell, Mérida Salvador, and Navea Amparo. "Oxidative Stress in Myopia." *Oxidative Medicine and Cellular Longevity* 2015 (April 1, 2015): 1-12. doi:10.1155/2015/750637.

2. Holden, Brien A., Timothy R. Fricke, David A. Wilson, Monica Jong, Kovin S. Naidoo, Padmaja Sankaridurg, Tien Y. Wong, Thomas J. Naduvilath, and Serge Resnikoff. "Global Prevalence of Myopia and High Myopia and Temporal Trends from 2000 through 2050." *Ophthalmology* 123, no. 5 (May 2016): 1036-042. doi:10.1016/j.ophtha.2016.01.006.

3. RSB, Director, and Director.rsb@anu.edu.au. "The Epidemic of Myopia in East and Southeast Asia." RSB. April 13, 2017. Accessed July 01, 2019. *https://biology.anu.edu.au/epidemic-myopia-east-and-southeast-asia*.

What is Myopia?

1. "Facts About Myopia." National Eye Institute. October 01, 2017. Accessed July 01, 2019. *https://nei.nih.gov/health/errors/myopia*.

2. "Nearsightedness: What Is Myopia?" American Academy of Ophthalmology. February 07, 2019. Accessed July 01, 2019. *https://www.aao.org/eye-health/diseases/myopia-nearsightedness*.

3. Aller, T. A. "Clinical Management of Progressive Myopia." *Eye* 28, no. 2 (2013): 147-53. doi:10.1038/eye.2013.259.

4. "Diopters, Aberration, and the Human Eye." Khan Academy. Accessed July 01, 2019. *https://www.khanacademy.org/science/physics/geometric-optics/lenses/v/diopters-aberration-and-the-human-eye*.

5. Bhardwaj, Veena. "Axial Length, Anterior Chamber Depth-A Study in Different Age Groups and Refractive Errors." *Journal of Clinical and Diagnostic Research*, 2013. doi:10.7860/jcdr/2013/7015.3473.

6. "Easily Check Your Diopter Numbers." Endmyopiaorg. Accessed July 01, 2019. *https://endmyopia.org/myopia-calculator-2/*.

7. Meng, Weihua, Jacqueline Butterworth, François Malecaze, and Patrick Calvas. "Axial Length of Myopia: A Review of Current Research." *Ophthalmologica* 225, no. 3 (October 2011): 127-34. doi:10.1159/000317072.

Habit #1. Change Beliefs and Empower Yourself

1. Zhu, Xiaoying, Neville A. Mcbrien, Earl L. Smith, David Troilo, and Josh Wallman. "Eyes in Various Species Can Shorten to Compensate for Myopic Defocus." *Investigative Ophthalmology & Visual Science* 54, no. 4 (2013): 2634. doi:10.1167/iovs.12-10514.

2. Read, Scott A., Michael J. Collins, and Beata P. Sander. "Human Optical Axial Length and Defocus." *Investigative Ophthalmology & Visual Science* 51, no. 12 (2010): 6262. doi:10.1167/iovs.10-5457.

3. Lipton, Bruce. "Think Beyond Your Genes - June 2018." Accessed July 01, 2019. *https://www.brucelipton.com/newsletter/think-beyond-your-genes-june-2018*.

4. Warner, Ellen. (1983). The role of belief in healing. *Canadian Medical Association* journal, 128(9), 1107–1109.

5. Sussman, Martin. *The Program for Better Vision: How to See Better in Minutes a Day without Glasses or Contacts!* Topsfield, MA: K-SEE Publications, 2005.

6. Hay, Louise L. *You Can Heal Your Life*. Carlsbad, CA: Hay House, 2017.

Habit #2. Caution the Quick Fix

1. Bates, William H. *The Bates Method for Better Eyesight without Glasses*. London: Thorsons, 2000.

2. Li, Shi-Ming, Shan-Shan Wu, Meng-Tian Kang, Ying Liu, Shu-Mei Jia, Si-Yuan Li, Si-Yan Zhan, Luo-Ru Liu, He Li, Wei Chen, Zhou Yang, Yun-Yun Sun, Ningli Wang, and Michel Millodot. "Atropine Slows Myopia Progression More in Asian Than White Children by Meta-analysis." *Optometry and Vision Science*, 2014, 1. doi:10.1097/opx.0000000000000178.

3. Marsh, Doug. *Restoring Your Eyesight: A Taoist Approach*. Rochester, VT: Healing Arts Press, 2007.

4. Arumugam, Baskar, Li-Fang Hung, Chi-Ho To, Brien Holden, and Earl L. Smith. "The Effects of Simultaneous Dual Focus Lenses on Refractive Development in Infant Monkeys." *Investigative Ophthalmology & Visual Science* 55, no. 11 (2014): 7423. doi:10.1167/iovs.14-14250.

5. Tse, Dennis Y., and Chi-Ho To. "Graded Competing Regional Myopic and Hyperopic Defocus Produce Summated Emmetropization Set Points in Chick." *Investigative Ophthalmology & Visual Science* 52, no. 11 (2011): 8056. doi:10.1167/iovs.10-5207.

6. Sun, Yun-Yun, Shi-Ming Li, Si-Yuan Li, Meng-Tian Kang, Luo-Ru Liu, Bo Meng, Feng-Ju Zhang, Michel Millodot, and Ningli Wang. "Effect of Uncorrection versus Full Correction on Myopia

Progression in 12-year-old Children." *Graefes Archive for Clinical and Experimental Ophthalmology* 255, no. 1 (2016): 189-95. doi:10.1007/ s00417-016-3529-1.

7. Chung, Kahmeng, Norhani Mohidin, and Daniel J. O'Leary. "Undercorrection of Myopia Enhances Rather than Inhibits Myopia Progression." *Vision Research* 42, no. 22 (2002): 2555-559. doi:10.1016/ s0042-6989(02)00258-4.

Habit #3. Examine Your Lifestyle

1. Francisco, Bosch-Morell, Mérida Salvador, and Navea Amparo. "Oxidative Stress in Myopia." *Oxidative Medicine and Cellular Longevity* 2015 (April 1, 2015): 1-12. doi:10.1155/2015/750637.

2. "Familial Aggregation and Prevalence of Myopia in the Framingham Offspring Eye Study." *Archives of Ophthalmology* 114, no. 3 (1996): 326. doi:10.1001/archopht.1996.01100130322017.

3. Morgan, Ian G., Kyoko Ohno-Matsui, and Seang-Mei Saw. "Myopia." The Lancet 379, no. 9827 (2012): 1739-748. doi:10.1016/ s0140-6736(12)60272-4.

4. Vitale, S et al. 2009. Increased prevalence of myopia in the United States between 1971-1972 and 1999-2004. *Arch Ophthalmol* 127(12): 1632-1639.

5. Holden, Brien A., Timothy R. Fricke, David A. Wilson, Monica Jong, Kovin S. Naidoo, Padmaja Sankaridurg, Tien Y. Wong, Thomas J. Naduvilath, and Serge Resnikoff. "Global Prevalence of Myopia and High Myopia and Temporal Trends from 2000 through 2050." *Ophthalmology* 123, no. 5 (2016): 1036-042. doi:10.1016/j.ophtha.2016.01.006.

6. Nelson, L.B. "Myopia, Lifestyle and Schooling in Students of Chinese Ethnicity in Singapore and Sydney." *Yearbook of Ophthalmology* 2009 (2009): 179. doi:10.1016/s0084-392x(09)79154-3.

7. "Health Risks of an Inactive Lifestyle." MedlinePlus. December 21, 2018. Accessed July 01, 2019. https://medlineplus.gov/healthrisksofaninactivelifestyle.html.

8. O'Donoghue, Lisa, Venediktos V. Kapetanankis, Julie F. McClelland, Nicola S. Logan, Christopher G. Owen, Kathryn J. Saunders, and Alicja R. Rudnicka. "Risk Factors for Childhood Myopia: Findings from the NICER Study." *Investigative Ophthalmology & Visual Science*. March 01, 2015. Accessed July 02, 2019. *https://iovs.arvojournals.org/article.aspx?articleid=2212924*

Habit #4. Eat Nutrient-Rich Diet

1. Bénédicte M.J. Merle, Johanna M. Colijn, Audrey Cougnard-Grégoire, Alexandra P.M. de Koning-Backus, Marie-Noëlle Delyfer, Jessica C.

Kiefte-de Jong, Magda Meester-Smoor, Catherine Féart, Timo Verzijden, Cécilia Samieri, Oscar H. Franco, Jean-François Korobelnik, Caroline C.W. Klaver, Cécile Delcourt, for the show EYE-RISK Consortium. "Mediterranean Diet and Incidence of Advanced Age-Related Macular Degeneration." *Ophthalmology* 126, no. 3 (2019): 381-390. doi: 10.1016/j.ophtha.2018.08.006

2. Francisco, Bosch-Morell, Mérida Salvador, and Navea Amparo. "Oxidative Stress in Myopia." *Oxidative Medicine and Cellular Longevity* 2015 (April 1, 2015): 1-12. doi:10.1155/2015/750637

3. Johnson, Elizabeth J. "The Role of Carotenoids in Human Health." *Nutrition in Clinical Care* 5, no. 2 (2002): 56-65. doi:10.1046/j.1523-5408.2002.00004.x.

4. Dimova, Svetlana, Peter H.m. Hoet, David Dinsdale, and Benoit Nemery. "Acetaminophen Decreases Intracellular Glutathione Levels and Modulates Cytokine Production in Human Alveolar Macrophages and Type II Pneumocytes in Vitro." *The International Journal of Biochemistry & Cell Biology* 37, no. 8 (2005): 1727-737. doi:10.1016/j.biocel.2005.03.005.

5. Seeram, Navindra P. "Berry Fruits for Cancer Prevention: Current Status and Future Prospects." *Journal of Agricultural and Food Chemistry* 56, no. 3 (2008): 630-35. doi:10.1021/jf072504n.

6. Huibi, Xu, Huang Kaixun, Gao Qiuhua, Zhu Yushan, and Han Xiuxian. "Prevention of Axial Elongation in Myopia by the Trace Element Zinc." *Biological Trace Element Research* 79, no. 1 (2001): 39-47. doi:10.1385/bter:79:1:39.

7. "Vitamins and Minerals." National Center for Complementary and Integrative Health. February 09, 2018. Accessed July 02, 2019. *https://nccih.nih. gov/health/vitamins*.

8. Brown, Nicholas A Phelps, Anthony J. Bron, John J. Harding, and Helen M. Dewar. "Nutrition Supplements and the Eye." *Eye* 12, no. 1 (1998): 127-33. doi:10.1038/eye.1998.21.

9. Akbaraly, Tasnime N., Eric J. Brunner, Jane E. Ferrie, Michael G. Marmot, Mika Kivimaki, and Archana Singh-Manoux. "Dietary Pattern and Depressive Symptoms in Middle Age." *British Journal of Psychiatry* 195, no. 5 (2009): 408-13. doi:10.1192/bjp.bp.108.058925.

10. Fiolet, Thibault, Bernard Srour, Laury Sellem, Emmanuelle Kesse-Guyot, Benjamin Allès, Caroline Méjean, Mélanie Deschasaux, Philippine Fassier, Paule Latino-Martel, Marie Beslay, Serge Hercberg, Céline Lavalette, Carlos A. Monteiro, Chantal Julia, and Mathilde Touvier. "Consumption of Ultra-processed Foods and Cancer Risk: Results from NutriNet-Santé Prospective Cohort." *Bmj*, 2018. doi:10.1136/bmj.k322.

11. "Q&A on the Carcinogenicity of the Consumption of Red Meat and Processed Meat." World Health Organization. May 17, 2016. Accessed July 02, 2019. *https://www.who.int/features/qa/cancer-red-meat/en/*.

12. Cordain, Loren, S. Boyd Eaton, Jennie Brand Miller, Staffan Lindeberg, and Clark Jensen. "An Evolutionary Analysis of the Aetiology and Pathogenesis of Juvenile-onset Myopia - Cordain - 2002 - Acta Ophthalmologica Scandinavica - Wiley Online Library." *Acta Ophthalmologica Scandinavica*. March 12, 2003. Accessed July 02, 2019. *https://onlinelibrary.wiley.com/doi/full/10.1034/j.1600-0420.2002.800203.x*.

13. Lane, B. C. "Calcium, Chromium, Protein, Sugar and Accommodation in Myopia." *SpringerLink*. January 01, 1981. Accessed July 02, 2019. *https://link.springer.com/chapter/10.1007/978-94-009-8662-6_21*.

Habit #5. Get Enough Sleep

1. Walker, Matthew P. *Why We Sleep: Unlocking the Power of Sleep and Dreams*. New York, NY: Scribner, an Imprint of Simon & Schuster, 2018.

2. Jee, Donghyun, Ian G. Morgan, and Eun Chul Kim. "Inverse Relationship between Sleep Duration and Myopia." *Acta Ophthalmologica* 94, no. 3 (2015). doi:10.1111/aos.12776.

3. Ayaki, Masahiko, Hidemasa Torii, Kazuo Tsubota, and Kazuno Negishi. "Decreased Sleep Quality in High Myopia Children." *Scientific Reports* 6, no. 1 (2016). doi:10.1038/srep33902.

4. Green, A., M. Cohen-Zion, A. Haim, and Y. Dagan. "Evening Light Exposure from Computer Screens Disrupts Sleep, Biological Rhythms and Attention Abilities." *Sleep Medicine* 40 (2017). doi:10.1016/j.sleep.2017.11.343.

Habit #6. Mind Your Posture

1. "The American Optometric Association's Clinical Practice Guide, Care of the Patient with Myopia." American Optometric Association. August 9, 1997. Reviewed February 2001, Reviewed 2006. Accessed July 02, 2019. *https://www.aoa.org/documents/optometrists/CPG-15.pdf.*

2. Pärssinen, Olavi, and Markku Kauppinen. "Associations of Reading Posture, Gaze Angle and Reading Distance with Myopia and Myopic Progression." *Acta Ophthalmologica* 94, no. 8 (2016): 775-79. doi:10.1111/aos.13148.

3. Bao, Jinhua, Björn Drobe, Yuwen Wang, Ke Chen, Eu Jin Seow, and Fan Lu. "Influence of Near Tasks on Posture in Myopic Chinese Schoolchildren." *Optometry and Vision Science* 92, no. 8 (2015): 908-15. doi:10.1097/opx.0000000000000658.

4. "Unexpected Link Between Posture and Your Eyes." Accessed July 02, 2019. *https://www.drbishop.com/ blog/unexpected-link-between-posture-and-your-eyes/*

5. Carney, Dana R., Amy J C Cuddy, and Andy J. Yap. "Power Posing: Brief Nonverbal Displays Affect Neuroendocrine Levels and Risk Tolerance." *Psychological Science*. October 2010. Accessed July 02, 2019. *https://www.ncbi.nlm.nih.gov/ pubmed/20855902*.

6. Cuddy, Amy. "Your Body Language May Shape Who You Are." TED. Accessed July 02, 2019. *https://www.ted.com/talks/amy_cuddy_your_body_ language_shapes_who_you_are*.

Habit #7. Practice 20-20-20

1. "Computers, Digital Devices and Eye Strain." American Academy of Ophthalmology. October 18, 2018. Accessed July 02, 2019. *https://www.aao.org/ eye-health/tips-prevention/computer-usage*.

2. "Time Flies: U.S. Adults Now Spend Nearly Half a Day Interacting with Media." Nielsen. Accessed July 02, 2019. *https://www.nielsen.com/us/en/ insights/article/2018/time-flies-us-adults-now- spend-nearly-half-a-day-interacting-with-media/*.

3. "Problems & Conditions." Digital Eye Strain | The Vision Council. Accessed July 02, 2019. *https:// www.thevisioncouncil.org/content/digital-eye-strain/ kids*

4. "Ergonomics Awareness Training for Workplace Design Engineers." *Applied Ergonomics* 22, no. 6 (1991): 416-17. doi:10.1016/0003-6870(91)90093-w.

5. Reddy, S. C., C. K. Low, Y. P. Lim, L. L. Low, F. Mardina, and M. P. Nursaleha. "Computer Vision Syndrome: A Study of Knowledge and Practices in University Students." *Nepalese Journal of Ophthalmology*: A Biannual Peer-reviewed Academic Journal of the Nepal Ophthalmic Society: NEPJOPH. 2013. Accessed July 02, 2019. *https://www.ncbi.nlm.nih.gov/pubmed/24172549*.

6. Sussman, Martin. *The Program for Better Vision: How to See Better in Minutes a Day without Glasses or Contacts!* Topsfield, MA: K-SEE Publications, 2005.

Habit #8. Do Your Eye Exercise

1. Lustig, Robert H. *Fat Chance: Beating the Odds against Sugar, Processed Food, Obesity, and Disease*. New York: Plume, 2014.

2. Lin, Zhong, Balamurali Vasudevan, Vishal Jhanji, Tie Ying Gao, Ning Li Wang, Qi Wang, Ji Wang, Kenneth J. Ciuffreda, and Yuan Bo Liang. "Eye Exercises of Acupoints: Their Impact on Refractive Error and Visual Symptoms in Chinese Urban Children." *BMC Complementary and Alternative Medicine* 13, no. 1 (2013). doi:10.1186/1472-6882-13-306.

3. Noto, Paula Di, Sorin Uta, and Joseph F. X. Desouza. "Eye Exercises Enhance Accuracy and Letter Recognition, but Not Reaction Time, in a Modified Rapid Serial Visual Presentation Task." *PLoS ONE* 8, no. 3 (2013). doi:10.1371/journal.pone.0059244.

4. Kang, Meng-Tian, Shi-Ming Li, Xiaoxia Peng, Lei Li, Anran Ran, Bo Meng, Yunyun Sun, Luo-Ru Liu, He Li, Michel Millodot, and Ningli Wang. "Chinese Eye Exercises and Myopia Development in School Age Children: A Nested Case-control Study." *Scientific Reports* 6, no. 1 (2016). doi:10.1038/srep28531.

5. Bates, William H. The Bates Method for Better Eyesight without Glasses. London: Thorsons, 2000.

6. Gardner, Benjamin, Phillippa Lally, and Jane Wardle. "Making Health Habitual: The Psychology of 'habit-formation' and General Practice." *British Journal of General Practice* 62, no. 605 (2012): 664-66. doi:10.3399/bjgp12x659466.

7. "Deepak Chopra's Eye Exercises." TruthWiki. February 28, 2017. Accessed July 02, 2019. *http://www.truthwiki.org/deepak_chopras_eye_exercises/*.

Habit #9. Learn How to Use Prescription Lenses

1. Walline, Jeffrey J., Amber Gaume, Lisa A. Jones, Marjorie J. Rah, Ruth E. Manny, David

A. Berntsen, Monica Chitkara, Ailene Kim, and Nicole Quinn. "Benefits of Contact Lens Wear for Children and Teens." *Eye & Contact Lens: Science & Clinical Practice* 33, no. 6, Part 1 of 2 (2007): 317-21. doi:10.1097/icl.0b013e31804f80fb.

2. Fateme Alipour, Saeed Khaheshi, Mahya Soleimanzadeh, Somayeh Heidarzadeh, Sepideh Heydarzadeh. *Journal of Ophthalmic and Vision Research*. 2017 Apr-Jun; 12(2): 193–204. doi: 10.4103/jovr.jovr_159_16.

3. Center for Devices and Radiological Health. "Contact Lens Risks." U.S. Food and Drug Administration. Accessed July 02, 2019. *https://www.fda.gov/ MedicalDevices/ProductsandMedicalProcedures/ HomeHealthandConsumer/ConsumerProducts/ ContactLenses/ucm062589.htm*.

4. Yun-Yun Sun, Shi-Ming Li, Feng-Ju Zhang Bo Meng, Michel Millodot, and Ningli Wang. "Effect of Uncorrection versus Full Correction on Myopia Progression in 12-year-old Children." *SpringerLink*. October 29, 2016. Accessed July 02, 2019. *https://link.springer.com/article/10.1007/ s00417-016-3529-1*.

Habit #10. Reduce Your Stress

1. Louise Katz and Kristoffer S. Berlin. "Psychological Stress in Childhood and Myopia Development."

Optometry & Visual Performance. (December 2014), 2(6) : 289-296. doi:10.1037/t51372-000.

2. Melanie J. Murphy Edwards, Agnes Hazi, Sheila G. Crewther; "Acute Psychosocial Stress Induces a Myopic Shift in Undergraduate Students." *Invest. Ophthalmol. Vis. Sci.* 2011;52(14):2841.

3. Moser, Jason S., Adrienne Dougherty, Whitney I. Mattson, Benjamin Katz, Tim P. Moran, Darwin Guevarra, Holly Shablack, Ozlem Ayduk, John Jonides, Marc G. Berman, and Ethan Kross. "Third-person Self-talk Facilitates Emotion Regulation without Engaging Cognitive Control: Converging Evidence from ERP and FMRI." *Scientific Reports* 7, no. 1 (2017). doi:10.1038/s41598-017-04047-3.

4. McGonigal, Kelly. "How to Make Stress Your Friend." TED. Accessed July 02, 2019. *https://www.ted.com/talks/kelly_mcgonigal_how_to_make_stress_your_friend?language=en.*

5. Orme-Johnson, D. "Medical Care Utilization and the Transcendental Meditation Program." *Psychosomatic Medicine* 49, no. 5 (1987): 493-507. doi:10.1097/00006842-198709000-00006.

6. Church, Dawson, Garret Yount, and Audrey J. Brooks. "The Effect of Emotional Freedom Techniques on Stress Biochemistry." *The Journal of Nervous and Mental Disease* 200, no. 10 (2012): 891-96. doi:10.1097/nmd.0b013e31826b9fc1.

Habit #11. Manage Your Emotions

1. Sussman, Martin. *The Program for Better Vision: How to See Better in Minutes a Day without Glasses or Contacts!* Topsfield, MA: K-SEE Publications, 2005.

2. Wu, Yin, Qinghua Ma, Hong-Peng Sun, Yong Xu, Mei-E Niu, and Chen-Wei Pan. "Myopia and Depressive Symptoms among Older Chinese Adults." *Plos One* 12, no. 5 (2017). doi:10.1371/journal.pone.0177613.

3. "5 Ways Stress Hurts Your Body, and What to Do About It." Psychology Today. Accessed July 02, 2019. *https://www.psychologytoday.com/us/blog/urban-survival/201505/5-ways-stress-hurts-your-body-and-what-do-about-it.*

4. Louise Katz and Kristoffer S. Berlin. "Psychological Stress in Childhood and Myopia Development." *Optometry & Visual Performance.* (December 2014), 2(6) : 289-296. doi:10.1037/t51372-000

5. Truman, Karol Kuhn. *Feelings Buried Alive Never Die.* Phoenix, AZ: Olympus Distributing, 2015.

6. Salovey, Peter, Alexander J. Rothman, Jerusha B. Detweiler, and Wayne T. Steward. "Emotional States and Physical Health." *American Psychologist* 55, no. 1 (2000): 110-21. doi:10.1037//0003-066x.55.1.110.

7. Carr, Brittany J. "The Science Behind Myopia." Webvision: The Organization of the Retina and

Visual System [Internet]. November 07, 2017. Accessed July 02, 2019. *https://www.ncbi.nlm.nih. gov/books/NBK470669/.*

8. Zhou, Xiangtian, Machelle T. Pardue, P. Michael Iuvone, and Jia Qu. "Dopamine Signaling and Myopia Development: What Are the Key Challenges." *Progress in Retinal and Eye Research* 61 (2017): 60-71. doi:10.1016/j. preteyeres.2017.06.003

Habit #12. Relax Your Mind and Eye Muscles

1. Arunthavaraja, Mathangi, Balamurali Vasudevan, and Kenneth J. Ciuffreda. "Nearwork-induced Transient Myopia (NITM) following Marked and Sustained, but Interrupted, Accommodation at near." *Ophthalmic and Physiological Optics* 30, no. 6 (2010): 766-75. doi:10.1111/j.1475-1313.2010.00787.x.

2. Carr, Brittany J. "The Science Behind Myopia." Webvision: The Organization of the Retina and Visual System [Internet]. November 07, 2017. Accessed July 02, 2019. *https://www.ncbi.nlm.nih. gov/books/NBK470669/.*

3. Walline, Jeffrey J., Kristina Lindsley, Satyanarayana S. Vedula, Susan A. Cotter, Donald O. Mutti, and J. Daniel Twelker. "Interventions to Slow Progression of Myopia in Children."

Cochrane Database of Systematic Reviews, 2011. doi:10.1002/14651858.cd004916.pub3.

4. Yam, Jason C., Yuning Jiang, Shu Min Tang, Antony K.p. Law, Joyce J. Chan, Emily Wong, Simon T. Ko, Alvin L. Young, Clement C. Tham, Li Jia Chen, and Chi Pui Pang. "Low-Concentration Atropine for Myopia Progression (LAMP) Study." *Ophthalmology* 126, no. 1 (2019): 113-24. doi:10.1016/j.ophtha.2018.05.029.

5. Chia, Audrey, Wei-Han Chua, Yin-Bun Cheung, Wan-Ling Wong, Anushia Lingham, Allan Fong, and Donald Tan. "Atropine for the Treatment of Childhood Myopia: Safety and Efficacy of 0.5%, 0.1%, and 0.01% Doses (Atropine for the Treatment of Myopia 2)." *Ophthalmology* 119, no. 2 (2012): 347-54. doi:10.1016/j.ophtha.2011.07.031.

6. Gong, Qianwen, Miroslaw Janowski, Mi Luo, Hong Wei, Bingjie Chen, Guoyuan Yang, and Longqian Liu. "Efficacy and Adverse Effects of Atropine in Childhood Myopia." *JAMA Ophthalmology* 135, no. 6 (2017): 624. doi:10.1001/jamaophthalmol.2017.1091.

7. Wu, Pei-Chang, Meng-Ni Chuang, Jessy Choi, Huan Chen, Grace Wu, Kyoko Ohno-Matsui, Jost B. Jonas, and Chui Ming Gemmy Cheung. "Update in Myopia and Treatment Strategy of Atropine Use in Myopia Control." *Eye* 33, no. 1 (2018): 3-13. doi:10.1038/s41433-018-0139-7.

Habit #13. Go Outdoors and Play

1. Carr, Brittany J. "The Science Behind Myopia." Webvision: The Organization of the Retina and Visual System [Internet]. November 07, 2017. Accessed July 02, 2019. *https://www.ncbi.nlm.nih. gov/books/NBK470669/*

2. Morgan, Ian G., Amanda N. French, Regan S. Ashby, Xinxing Guo, Xiaohu Ding, Mingguang He, and Kathryn A. Rose. "The Epidemics of Myopia: Aetiology and Prevention." *Progress in Retinal and Eye Research* 62 (2018): 134-49. doi:10.1016/j. preteyeres.2017.09.004.

3. Tosini, Gianluca, Ian Ferguson, and Kazuo Tsubota. "Effects of Blue Light on the Circadian System and Eye Physiology." *Molecular Vision*. January 24, 2016. Accessed July 02, 2019. *https://www.ncbi. nlm.nih.gov/pubmed/26900325*.

4. Pandita, Aaakash, Deepak Sharma, Dharti Pandita, Smita Pawar, Avinash Kaul, and Mir Tariq. "Childhood Obesity: Prevention Is Better than Cure." *Diabetes, Metabolic Syndrome and Obesity: Targets and Therapy*, 2016, 83. doi:10.2147/dmso. s90783.

5. Jin, Ju-Xiang, Wen-Juan Hua, Xuan Jiang, Xiao-Yan Wu, Ji-Wen Yang, Guo-Peng Gao, Yun Fang, Chen-Lu Pei, Song Wang, Jie-Zheng Zhang, Li-Ming Tao, and Fang-Biao Tao. "Effect of Outdoor Activity on Myopia Onset and Progression in

School-aged Children in Northeast China: The Sujiatun Eye Care Study." *BMC Ophthalmology* 15, no. 1 (2015). doi:10.1186/s12886-015-0052-9.

6. Rose, K.A., D. Robaei, A. Kifley, W. Smith, P. Mitchell, and I.G. Morgan. "Near–Work and Outdoor Activities and the Prevalence of Myopia in Australian School Students Aged 12–13 Years: The Sydney Myopia Study." *Investigative Ophthalmology & Visual Science*. Vol.47, 5453. (May 01, 2006).

7. Morgan, Ian G. "Myopia Prevention and Outdoor Light Intensity in a School-based Cluster Randomized Trial." *Ophthalmology* 125, no. 8 (2018): 1251-252. doi:10.1016/j. ophtha.2018.04.016.

8. Stockman, J.a. "Outdoor Activity Reduces the Prevalence of Myopia in Children." *Yearbook of Pediatrics* 2010 (2010): 505-07. doi:10.1016/ s0084-3954(09)79489-8.

9. Mcknight, Charlotte M., Justin C. Sherwin, Seyhan Yazar, Hannah Forward, Alex X. Tan, Alex W. Hewitt, Craig E. Pennell, Ian L. Mcallister, Terri L. Young, Minas T. Coroneo, and David A. Mackey. "Myopia in Young Adults Is Inversely Related to an Objective Marker of Ocular Sun Exposure: The Western Australian Raine Cohort Study." *American Journal of Ophthalmology* 158, no. 5 (2014). doi:10.1016/j.ajo.2014.07.033.

10. Zhou, Xiangtian, Machelle T. Pardue, P. Michael Iuvone, and Jia Qu. "Dopamine Signaling and Myopia Development: What Are the Key Challenges." *Progress in Retinal and Eye Research* 61 (2017): 60-71. doi:10.1016/j. preteyeres.2017.06.003.

11. Ashby, Regan S., and Frank Schaeffel. "The Effect of Bright Light on Lens Compensation in Chicks." *Investigative Ophthalmology & Visual Science* 51, no. 10 (2010): 5247. doi:10.1167/iovs.09-4689.

12. Smith, Earl L., Li-Fang Hung, Baskar Arumugam, and Juan Huang. "Negative Lens–Induced Myopia in Infant Monkeys: Effects of High Ambient Lighting." *Investigative Ophthalmology & Visual Science* 54, no. 4 (2013): 2959. doi:10.1167/ iovs.13-11713.

13. Smith, Earl L., Li-Fang Hung, and Juan Huang. "Protective Effects of High Ambient Lighting on the Development of Form-Deprivation Myopia in Rhesus Monkeys." *Investigative Ophthalmology & Visual Science* 53, no. 1 (2012): 421. doi:10.1167/ iovs.11-8652.

14. Louv, Richard. *Last Child in the Woods: Saving Our Children from Nature-Deficit Disorder*. London: Atlantic Books, 2013.

15. Wu, Pei-Chang, Chia-Ling Tsai, Hsiang-Lin Wu, Yi-Hsin Yang, and Hsi-Kung Kuo. "Outdoor Activity during Class Recess Reduces Myopia Onset and

Progression in School Children." *Ophthalmology* 120, no. 5 (2013): 1080-085. doi:10.1016/j. ophtha.2012.11.009.

16. Dolgin, Elie. "The Myopia Boom." *Nature* 519, no. 7543 (2015): 276-78. doi:10.1038/519276a.

Habit #14: Control Indoor Lighting

1. Landis, Erica G., Victoria Yang, Dillon M. Brown, Machelle T. Pardue, and Scott A. Read. "Dim Light Exposure and Myopia in Children." *Investigative Ophthalmology & Visual Science* 59, no. 12 (2018): 4804. doi:10.1167/iovs.18-24415.

2. Read, Scott A., Michael J. Collins, and Stephen J. Vincent. "Light Exposure and Physical Activity in Myopic and Emmetropic Children." *Optometry and Vision Science*, 2014, 1. doi:10.1097/ opx.0000000000000160.

3. Morgan, Ian G. "Myopia Prevention and Outdoor Light Intensity in a School-based Cluster Randomized Trial." *Ophthalmology* 125, no. 8 (2018): 1251-252. doi:10.1016/j. ophtha.2018.04.016.

4. Wu, Pei-Chang, Chia-Ling Tsai, Hsiang-Lin Wu, Yi-Hsin Yang, and Hsi-Kung Kuo. "Outdoor Activity during Class Recess Reduces Myopia Onset and Progression in School Children." *Ophthalmology* 120, no. 5 (2013): 1080-085. doi:10.1016/j. ophtha.2012.11.009.

5. Read, Scott A., Michael J. Collins, and Stephen J. Vincent. "Light Exposure and Eye Growth in Childhood." *Investigative Ophthalmology & Visual Science* 56, no. 11 (2015): 6779. doi:10.1167/iovs.14-15978.

6. Ashby, Regan, Arne Ohlendorf, and Frank Schaeffel. "The Effect of Ambient Illuminance on the Development of Deprivation Myopia in Chicks." *Investigative Ophthalmology & Visual Science* 50, no. 11 (2009): 5348. doi:10.1167/iovs.09-3419.

7. Smith, Earl L., Li-Fang Hung, Baskar Arumugam, and Juan Huang. "Negative Lens–Induced Myopia in Infant Monkeys: Effects of High Ambient Lighting." *Investigative Ophthalmology & Visual Science* 54, no. 4 (2013): 2959. doi:10.1167/iovs.13-11713.

8. Smith, Earl L., Li-Fang Hung, and Juan Huang. "Protective Effects of High Ambient Lighting on the Development of Form-Deprivation Myopia in Rhesus Monkeys." *Investigative Ophthalmology & Visual Science* 53, no. 1 (2012): 421. doi:10.1167/iovs.11-8652.

9. Zhou, Zhongqiang, Tingting Chen, Mengrui Wang, Ling Jin, Yongyi Zhao, Shangji Chen, Congyao Wang, Guoshan Zhang, Qilin Wang, Qiaoming Deng, Yubo Liu, Ian G. Morgan, Mingguang He, Yizhi Liu, and Nathan Congdon. "Pilot Study of a Novel Classroom Designed to Prevent Myopia by

Increasing Children's Exposure to Outdoor Light."
Plos One 12, no. 7 (2017). doi:10.1371/journal.
pone.0181772.

10. "Myopia Research: From the Margins to
the Mainstream." American Academy of
Ophthalmology. October 30, 2015. Accessed July
02, 2019. *https://www.aao.org/eyenet/article/
myopia-research-from-margins-to-mainstream*.

11. "Light-emitting-diode Induced Retinal Damage and
Its Wavelength Dependency in Vivo." *International
Journal of Ophthalmology*, 2017. doi:10.18240/
ijo.2017.02.03.

12. Moon, Jiyoung, Jieun Yun, Yeo Dae, Hye Yong
Chu, Myung Yeol Lee, Chang Woo Lee, Young-
Shin Kwak Soo Jin Oh, Young Pyo Jang, and Jong
Soon Kang. 2017. "Blue Light Effect on Retinal
Pigment Epithelial Cells by Display Devices."
Integrative Biology. The Royal Society of Chemistry.
March 21, 2017. *https://pubs.rsc.org/en/Content/
ArticleLanding/2017/IB/c7ib00032d#!divAbstract*.

13. Wright, Helen R., and Leon C. Lack. 2001.
"Effect of Light Wavelength On Suppression
And Phase Delay Of The Melatonin Rhythm."
Chronobiology International 18 (5): 801–8. *https://
doi.org/10.1081/cbi-100107515*.

Habit #15: Remove the Nightlight in the Bedroom

1. Quinn, Graham E., Chai H. Shin, Maureen G. Maguire, and Richard A. Stone. 1999. "Myopia and Ambient Lighting at Night." *Nature* 399 (6732): 113–14. *https://doi.org/10.1038/20094.*

2. Gwiazda, J., E. Ong, R. Held, and F. Thorn. 2000. "Myopia and Ambient Night-Time Lighting." *Nature* 404 (6774): 144–44. *https://doi.org/10.1038/35004663.*

3. Ayaki, Masahiko, Hidemasa Torii, Kazuo Tsubota, and Kazuno Negishi. 2016. "Decreased Sleep Quality in High Myopia Children." *Scientific Reports* 6 (1). *https://doi.org/10.1038/srep33902.*

4. Wright, Helen R., and Leon C. Lack. 2001. "Effect of Light Wavelength On Suppression And Phase Delay Of The Melatonin Rhythm." *Chronobiology International* 18 (5): 801–8. *https://doi.org/10.1081/cbi-100107515.*

5. Wright, Helen R., Leon C. Lack, and David J. Kennaway. 2004. "Differential Effects of Light Wavelength in Phase Advancing the Melatonin Rhythm." *Journal of Pineal Research* 36 (2): 140–44. *https://doi.org/10.1046/j.1600-079x.2003.00108.x.*

6. Lockley, Steven W., George C. Brainard, and Charles A. Czeisler. 2003. "High Sensitivity of the Human Circadian Melatonin Rhythm to Resetting by Short Wavelength Light." *The Journal of Clinical*

Endocrinology & Metabolism 88 (9): 4502–. *https:// doi.org/10.1210/jc.2003-030570.*

7. Ockwell-Smith, Sarah, and Sarah Ockwell-Smith. 2017. "Why Your Child's Night Light Is Ruining Their Sleep." HuffPost UK. HuffPost UK. March 31, 2017. *https://www.huffingtonpost.co.uk/sarah-ockwellsmith/night-light-children_b_9558914. html?guccounter=2.*

8. Walker, Matthew P. 2018. *Why We Sleep: Unlocking the Power of Sleep and Dreams.* New York, NY: Scribner, an imprint of Simon & Schuster, Inc.

9. Muraskas, Jonathan, and Kayhan Parsi. 2008. "The Cost of Saving the Tiniest Lives: NICUs versus Prevention." Journal of Ethics | American Medical Association. American Medical Association. October 1, 2008. *https://journalofethics.ama-assn. org/article/cost-saving-tiniest-lives-nicus-versus-prevention/2008-10.*

10. Klass, Perri. 2018. "To Help Children Sleep, Go Dark." The New York Times. The New York Times. March 5, 2018. *https://www.nytimes. com/2018/03/05/well/family/children-sleep-light-melatonin.html.*

Habit #16: Hang a Snellen Chart

1. Bates, William H. 2000. *The Bates Method for Better Eyesight without Glasses.* London: Thorsons.

2. Bates, William H. August 30, 1913. Myopia Prevention by Teachers. *American Journal of Ophthalmology*, Volumes 29-30.

Habit #17: Make Vision Health Habitual

1. Duhigg, Charles. 2014. *The Power of Habit: Why We Do What We Do in Life and Business*. Toronto: Anchor Canada.

2. Lally, Phillippa, Cornelia H. M. Van Jaarsveld, Henry W. W. Potts, and Jane Wardle. 2009. "How Are Habits Formed: Modelling Habit Formation in the Real World." *European Journal of Social Psychology* 40 (6): 998–1009. *https://doi.org/10.1002/ejsp.674*.

3. Clear, James. 2018. *Atomic Habits: Tiny Changes, Remarkable Results: An Easy & Proven Way to Build Good Habits & Break Bad Ones*. New York: Avery, an imprint of Penguin Random House.

4. Zylbermann, R, D Landau, and D Berson. 1993. "The Influence of Study Habits on Myopia in Jewish Teenagers." *Journal of Pediatric Ophthalmology and Strabismus*. U.S. National Library of Medicine. 1993 Sep-Oct;30(5):319-22. *https://www.ncbi.nlm.nih.gov/pubmed/8254449*.

5. Gardner, Benjamin, Phillippa Lally, and Jane Wardle. 2012. "Making Health Habitual: The Psychology of 'Habit-Formation' and General Practice." British Journal of General Practice

62 (605): 664–66. *https://doi.org/10.3399/ bjgp12x659466*.

Habit #18: SAVERS Morning Routine

1. Elrod, Hal. 2013. *The Miracle Morning. the Not-so-Obvious Secret Guaranteed to Transform Your Life before 8 AM*. Self-Published: Hal Elrod.

2. "Free Positive Affirmations." n.d. Free Affirmations Free Positive Affirmations. Accessed July 3, 2019. *https://www.freeaffirmations.org/*.

Habit #19: PEACE Daily Routine

1. Ma, Xiao, Zi-Qi Yue, Zhu-Qing Gong, Hong Zhang, Nai-Yue Duan, Yu-Tong Shi, Gao-Xia Wei, and You-Fa Li. 2017. "The Effect of Diaphragmatic Breathing on Attention, Negative Affect and Stress in Healthy Adults." *Frontiers in Psychology* 8. *https://doi.org/10.3389/fpsyg.2017.00874*.

2. Kraft, Tara L., and Sarah D. Pressman. 2012. "Grin and Bear It." *Psychological Science* 23 (11): 1372–78. *https://doi.org/10.1177/0956797612445312*.

3. "It's Official—Spending Time Outside Is Good for You." 2018. ScienceDaily. ScienceDaily. July 6, 2018. *https://www.sciencedaily.com/ releases/2018/07/180706102842.htm*.

Habit #20: DREAM Evening Routine

1. "Affirmations for Improving Eyesight."
   n.d. SelfGrowth.com. Accessed July 2,
   2019. *https://www.selfgrowth.com/articles/ affirmations-for-improving-eyesight*.

2. Ong, Jason C., Rachel Manber, Zindel Segal,
   Yinglin Xia, Shauna Shapiro, and James K. Wyatt.
   "A Randomized Controlled Trial of Mindfulness
   Meditation for Chronic Insomnia." *Sleep* 37, no. 9
   (2014): 1553-563. doi:10.5665/sleep.4010.

ACKNOWLEDGEMENTS

THANK YOU, FIRST AND foremost, my readers for taking the time to read this book. I am delighted that you are starting this journey towards better vision.

Seth Godin, the famous author, entrepreneur, and teacher said, "All I can do is borrow. I don't know of any purely original ideas, ones that arrive from the sky on a bolt of lightning. And if I borrow great ideas and recombine them in interesting ways, perhaps I can contribute something to the next person." In this book, I have borrowed ideas from hundreds of scientific researchers and book authors who made their great work available. I am standing on their shoulders.

My book idea comes from James Altucher, my favorite writer, podcaster, and entrepreneur, who created his 2019 Book Writing Challenge—to write a short book about (scientifically proven) habits and upload it to Amazon. The idea stuck with me during Christmas holiday when I was choosing among a couple of book ideas. It instantly became my new year resolution—to publish this book (which I have contemplated for five years) by summertime.

My dear husband, William, is the wind beneath my wings—thank you for supporting me to do what my heart calls me to do. I want to thank my beautiful children who inspired me to write this book and practiced what I write here. I also want to thank my extended family and friends who shared their personal stories and their journey with me.

Thank you, Katie Chambers, my editor, for your knowledge, patience, and wisdom. My cover designer, Danijela Mijailovic, my interior designer, Lazar Kackarovski, thank you for your creativity and professional work.

I want to thank the team from the Self-Publishing School tribe: Scott Allan, Chandler Bolt, Sean Sumner, and the wonderful mastermind community. You taught me, supported me, and pushed and pulled me when I needed a boost.

I want to thank my launch team who gave me precious ideas and feedback along the way. To everyone who agreed to help promote and share this book in some way, shape, or form—thank you for giving this book life!

About Aileen Yi Fan

AILEEN YI FAN IS a committed lifelong learner and an advocate for change. She holds a bachelor's degree in biomedical engineering and a master's degree in business administration. As the owner of a boutique marketing and PR agency serving small businesses, she believes that she teaches what she needs to learn the most. This book is a perfect example of her invest-learn-teach formula. Aileen loves sharing her life experiences, challenges, and lessons so like-minded people can gather, learn, and inspire each other. Her two beautiful children, Ian and Amy, inspire her to be the best version of herself, and to make a little progress every day—physically, emotionally, intellectually, and spiritually.

URGENT PLEA!

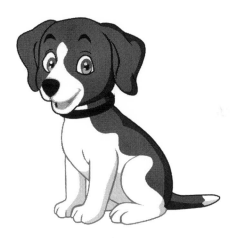

THANK YOU FOR READING MY BOOK!

I really appreciate all of your feedback, and I love hearing what you have to say.

I need your valuable input to make the next version of this book and my future books better.

Please leave me a helpful review on Amazon letting me know what you think of the book.

Thank you so much!

Aileen

Made in the USA
Columbia, SC
21 December 2019

85660014R00109